PARAMEDIC

SURVIVAL GUIDE

PARAMEDIC

SURVIVAL GUIDE

PETER A. DIPRIMA, JR, EMT-P

Instructor, Suffolk County Emergency Medical Services
Paramedic/Firefighter
Lakeland Fire Department
Suffolk County, New York

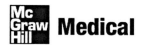

New York   Chicago   San Francisco   Lisbon   London   Madrid   Mexico City
Milan   New Delhi   San Juan   Seoul   Singapore   Sydney   Toronto

Paramedic Survival Guide

1 2 3 4 5 6 7 8 9 0   DOC/DOC   16 15 14 13 12

ISBN 978-0-07-176929-7
MHID 0-07-176929-3

This book was set in Minion Pro by Cenveo Publisher Services.
The editors were Kirsten Funk and Robert Pancotti.
The production supervisor was Sherri Souffrance.
Project management was provided by Rohini Deb, Cenveo Publisher Services.
The text designer was Alan Barnett.
Cover photograph © Getty Images.
RR Donnelley was printer and binder.

This book is printed on acid-free paper.

Library of Congress Cataloging-in-Publication Data

DiPrima, Peter A.
    Paramedic survival guide / Peter A. DiPrima Jr.
        p. ; cm.
    Includes bibliographical references and index.
    ISBN-13: 978-0-07-176929-7 (pbk. : alk. paper)
    ISBN-10: 0-07-176929-3 (pbk. : alk. paper)
    I. Title. [DNLM: 1. Emergency Medical Technicians.   2. Professional Practice.
3. Vocational Guidance. W 21.5]
    616.02'5092—dc23
                                                                2011044400

McGraw-Hill books are available at special quantity discounts to use as premiums and sales promotions, or for use in corporate training programs. To contact a representative, please e-mail us at bulksales@mcgraw-hill.com.

To my family
(Sue, Gabby, Jack, Mom and Dad DiPrima, and Sparling).
Thank you for believing in me.
Please do not ever doubt my dedication and love for you.

CONTENTS

CONTRIBUTORS

Louis Brand, BS, NREMT-P

Port Jefferson EMS
Setauket Fire and Rescue
Setauket, New York

Thomas E. Hoar III, BA, EMT-P

Port Jefferson EMS
Brentwood EMS
Setauket Fire and Rescue
Setauket New York

Daniel E. Meisels, MPA, EMT-P, CHEP

Director, EMS Program
University of Massachusetts Memorial Medical Center
Worcester, Massachusetts
Faculty, Center for Excellence in Emergency Preparedness Education (CEEPET)
University of Massachusetts Medical School
Worcester, Massachusetts
EMT-Paramedic
New York-Presbyterian Hospital EMS
New York, New York

Christopher VanHouten, EMT-P

New York-Presbyterian Hospital EMS
New York, New York

REVIEWERS

Angel Aviles
Paramedic Student
New Haven Sponsor
  Hospital
New Haven, Connecticut
Class of 2012

Joe Bart, DO, EMT-P/T
Department of Emergency
  Medicine
The State University of New York
Buffalo, New York

James F. Goss, MHA, MICP
Assistant Professor
Loma Linda University
School of Allied Health
  Professions
Emergency Medical Care
  Program
Loma Linda, California

Scott C. Jones, MBA, EMT-P
Associate Professor
Paramedic Academy
Victor Valley College
Victorville, California

Brian Kern, MD, EMT
Department of Emergency
  Medicine
Detroit Receiving Hospital
Detroit Medical Center
Wayne State University
Detroit, Michigan

Richard A. Nydam, EMT-P
Training Coordinator
University of Massachusetts Memorial
Healthcare
Worcester EMS
Worcester, Massachusetts;
Adjunct Faculty, Clinical Coordinator
Quinsigamond Community College
Paramedic Training Program
Worcester, Massachusetts

David Pecoraro, BS, EMT-P
New Haven Sponsor Hospital
New Haven, Connecticut

Brittany Selvaggi
Paramedic Student
New Haven Sponsor Hospital
New Haven, Connecticut
Class of 2011

Oliver Tatom
Paramedic Student
New Haven Sponsor Hospital
New Haven, Connecticut
Class of 2011

**Jorge D. Yarzebski, BA, NREMT-P,
CCEMT-P**
University of Massachusetts Medical School
Office of Continuing Education
University of Massachusetts Memorial
Healthcare
Worcester EMS
Worcester, Massachusetts

PREFACE

Despite rigorous medical education and training, are new paramedics equipped to handle all situations they may face? Over the course of our careers as emergency medical technicians and paramedics, we will encounter a remarkable number of scenarios not covered by formal education and training. Some are common and others are unusual. Some are life threatening and others are not. However, all are important and potentially challenging. Whenever the scenarios occur, people assume that you can and will be able to handle them just because you are or will be a paramedic!

Throughout the chapters of this book, I hope to fill some of the gaps in education and training, as well as help you with the who, what, where, and when of getting your career started. Paramedics typically have a driving need to feel knowledgeable and in control, even if their insides are spinning out of control. This book provides valuable tidbits of information that others around you may not know or have gained only through years of experience. Having such knowledge is empowering and fulfilling and will help you become a confident, respected, and important source of information and experience to others. Medicine, or more specifically paramedicine, is an ever-growing and changing field of science. It is sometimes difficult to represent text that is completely current upon publication. There are many ways to perform different skills and assessments that sometimes require the paramedic to think outside the box. So dive in and take your knowledge to another level. I hope you enjoy the book.

Experientia docet—Experience is the best teacher!

Peter A. DiPrima, Jr,
EMT-Paramedic/CIC

ACKNOWLEDGMENTS

I would like to extend my heartfelt gratitude to my past and present supervisors (Jack Delaney, Mike Timo, and Dr. Scott Coyne) and instructors whom I have been gratefully blessed to work with; you have made me believe that I have so much strength and courage to persevere. You were tolerant and determined to see me through. You were great motivators and I aspire to emulate you.

Finally, I would like to thank all of my colleagues who assisted, encouraged, and contributed to this book.

—PAD

EMT OATH

Be it pledged as an Emergency Medical Technician, I will honor the physical and judicial laws of God and man.

I will follow that regimen which, according to my ability and judgment, I consider for the benefit of patients and abstain from whatever is deleterious and mischievous, nor shall I suggest any such counsel.

Into whatever homes I enter, I will go into them for the benefit of only the sick and injured, never revealing what I see or hear in the lives of men unless required by law.

I shall also share my medical knowledge with those who may benefit from what I have learned.

I will serve unselfishly and continuously in order to help make a better world for all mankind.

While I continue to keep this oath unviolated, may it be granted to me to enjoy life, and the practice of the art, respected by all men, in all times.

Should I trespass or violate this oath, may the reverse be my lot.

So help me God.

Written by: Charles Gillespie, MD
Adopted by the National Association of EMTs
http://www.naemt.org

CODE OF ETHICS

Professional status as an Emergency Medical Technician and Emergency Medical Technician-Paramedic is maintained and enriched by the willingness of the individual practitioner to accept and fulfill obligations to society, other medical professionals, and the profession of Emergency Medical Technician. As an Emergency Medical Technician-Paramedic, I solemnly pledge myself to the following code of professional ethics:

A fundamental responsibility of the Emergency Medical Technician is to conserve life, to alleviate suffering, to promote health, to do no harm, and to encourage the quality and equal availability of emergency medical care.

The Emergency Medical Technician provides services based on human need, with respect for human dignity, unrestricted by consideration of nationality, race creed, color, or status.

The Emergency Medical Technician does not use professional knowledge and skills in any enterprise detrimental to the public well being.

The Emergency Medical Technician respects and holds in confidence all information of a confidential nature obtained in the course of professional work unless required by law to divulge such information.

The Emergency Medical Technician, as a citizen, understands and upholds the law and performs the duties of citizenship; as a professional, the Emergency Medical Technician has the never-ending responsibility to work with concerned citizens and other health care professionals in promoting a high standard of emergency medical care to all people.

The Emergency Medical Technician shall maintain professional competence and demonstrate concern for the competence of other members of the Emergency Medical Services health care team.

An Emergency Medical Technician assumes responsibility in defining and upholding standards of professional practice and education.

The Emergency Medical Technician assumes responsibility for individual professional actions and judgment, both in dependent and independent emergency functions, and knows and upholds the laws which affect the practice of the Emergency Medical Technician.

An Emergency Medical Technician has the responsibility to be aware of and participate in matters of legislation affecting the Emergency Medical Service System.

The Emergency Medical Technician, or groups of Emergency Medical Technicians, who advertise professional service, do so in conformity with the dignity of the profession.

The Emergency Medical Technician has an obligation to protect the public by not delegating to a person less qualified, any service which requires the professional competence of an Emergency Medical Technician

The Emergency Medical Technician will work harmoniously with and sustain confidence in Emergency Medical Technician associates, the nurses, the physicians, and other members of the Emergency Medical Services health care team.

The Emergency Medical Technician refuses to participate in unethical procedures, and assumes the responsibility to expose incompetence or unethical conduct of others to the appropriate authority in a proper and professional manner.

Written by: Charles Gillespie, MD
Adopted by the National Association of EMTs
http://www.naemt.org

INTRODUCTION

So paramedic school is over and rotations and lectures are done. No more classes, right? Well the real answer is, No! Medicine is an evolving science and it changes as much as I change my … well, I won't go there. What I am really saying is taking a little breather after your initial training is complete is much needed, and definitely acceptable. But your career is just starting and continual learning as a paramedic shouldn't stop. There are many opportunities available across the United States and abroad that will allow you to make a decent salary right out of paramedic school. (According to payscale.com, and depending on where you plan to work, salaries range from $24.50 to $31.21 per hour in New York City compared to Phoenix, Arizona, which has an average starting salary of $13.07 to $16.21 per hour.[1]) Each state has its own requirements for paramedic education and training, and to some extent, salaries will be determined on a state-by-state basis. In a comparison of paramedic salaries by state, New York offers higher salaries than many other states. Measuring the salary of paramedics by city reveals that paramedics in Chicago and Los Angeles also tend to earn higher salaries. If you are considering relocating, you may want to find out how far the salary of a paramedic will go in different areas.

As salaries vary from state to state, so do the educational requirements for paramedics. In the United States, the licensing or certification of pre-hospital emergency medical providers and oversight of emergency medical services are governed at the state level. Each state is free to add or subtract levels as each state sees fit. Therefore, due to differing needs and system development paths, the levels, education requirements, and scope of practice of pre-hospital providers vary from state to state. Although primary management and regulation of pre-hospital providers are at the state level, the federal government sets forth minimum requirements for EMT-Basics and EMT-Paramedics.

There isn't a day that goes by when I am working as a paramedic that I realize how much there is I can still learn. I guess that could be a book in itself. I hope this book guides you, the new paramedic, and gives the upper hand on a solid career in EMS. I will share some of my experiences, both good and bad, and hopefully reinforce a passion in a profession that is making new grounds, even as I write. To have a decent understanding on what or how we evolved, you need to have a brief history lesson. Again, you need to understand that paramedicine is relatively new as we know it. So sit back, enjoy yourself, and really know that your accomplishment of completing the paramedic course successfully is truly a great feat. Once you get bitten by the EMS bug, it's all over. I look back at my career as a paramedic and can say without any hesitation that it is the most rewarding and self-fulfilling career; I wouldn't change anything.

---

1   Payscale.com. Accessed June 20, 2010.

CHAPTER 1

EVOLUTION OF THE EMERGENCY MEDICAL SERVICES AND THE MAKING OF "PARAMEDICINE"

INTRODUCTION

In order for you to know where you are going, it helps to have an understanding of where you came from. Throughout the evolution of paramedicine, there has always been an ongoing association with military conflict. One of the first indications of a formal process for managing injured people dates back to the Imperial Legions of Rome, where aging centurions who were no longer able to fight were tasked with organizing the removal of the wounded from the battlefield and providing some form of care. Such individuals, though not physicians, were probably among the world's earliest surgeons, suturing wounds and performing amputations, not through training, but by default. This trend would continue throughout the Crusades, with the Knights Hospitallers of the Sovereign Order of St. John of Jerusalem, known throughout the Commonwealth of Nations today as St. John Ambulance, filling a similar function. Their motto to this day is "Pro fide. Pro utilitate hominum." or "For faith and in the service of humanity."[1]

The first vehicle that was specifically designed as an ambulance was created during the Napoleonic Wars. It was called the Ambulance Volante,

---

1   Knights Hospitallers of the Sovereign Order of St. John of Jerusalem. Our History. 2009. Available at: http://www.theknightshospitallers.org/history.php. Accessed June 23, 2010.

or "Flying Ambulance." Created by Napoleon's Chief Surgeon, Dominique Jean Larrey, the flying ambulances were horse-drawn wagons that were used to quickly collect and carry the wounded from the battlefield to base hospitals. Larrey described this concept in minute detail in a report from the Italian Campaign of 1797. It consisted of a system of transport of medical supplies and supporting personnel, including a doctor, a quartermaster, a noncommissioned officer, a drummer boy (who carried the bandages), and 24 infantrymen. The flying ambulances were a success, and this idea was subsequently taken up by other armies. Even in the harsh desert terrain, his flying ambulances would collect the wounded in less than 15 minutes[2]—pretty good response time!

The evolution of the ambulance took yet another turn during the American Civil War where ambulance wagons were too few, often late, and driven by civilians. Ambulance wagons were specially designed for the transport of sick and wounded but had not been used in the U.S. military until a year or so before the outbreak of the War of the Rebellion. Transport carts, army wagons, ox teams, or anything that could be made available for that purpose had been employed. In April 1777, during the War of Independence, the U.S. Congress passed a bill "devising ways and means for preserving the health of the troops," which contained the following paragraph: "That a suitable number of covered and other wagons, litters, and other necessaries for removing the sick and wounded, shall be supplied by the Quartermaster or Deputy Quartermaster General; and in case of their deficiency, by the Director or Deputy Director General." There is no record that such vehicles were supplied.

During the war with Great Britain, in 1812 to 1814, evidently there were no ambulance wagons in the U.S. Army; in his report of that campaign, Surgeon James Mann is found to make the request that "to facilitate the movement of the hospital department attached to an army, it should be furnished with a number of wagons and teams, so as not to be immediately dependent on the Quartermaster's Department, when requisite either to take the wounded from the field of battle, or transport the sick in case of a retrograde march, or remove invalids after having recovered from wounds to a remote hospital. The flying machines called *volant*, drawn by horses (an improvement of Larrey, Chief Surgeon of the French army), are useful in open countries, where a corps is assigned to accompany them on the field of battle, upon Larrey's plan." In February of 1814, the same author documents that he transported 450 sick men from

2   Skandalakis PN, Lainas P, Zoras O, Skandalakis JE, Mirilas P. "To Afford the Wounded Speedy Assistance": Dominique Jean Larrey and Napoleon. *World J Surg.* 2006;30:1392–1399. DOI: 10.1007/s00268-005-0436-8.

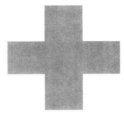

FIGURE 1-1. Protective signs are symbols to be used during an armed conflict to mark persons and objects under the protection of various treaties of international humanitarian law (IHL). An example of this would be Universal Red Cross.

Malone to Plattsburgh and Burlington, a distance of 70 miles, in sleighs, losing six patients by death. In 1838, during the Florida war, ambulance wagons are mentioned by Surgeon R.S. Satterlee, U.S.A., Medical Director south of Withlacoochee, in a report from Fort Brooke, Tampa Bay, dated January 5: "I found the ambulances very serviceable, but as some of the wounded could not be transported in them, on account of the roughness of the road, between thirty and forty of them were brought a part of the way on litters between two horses." Surgeon Satterlee probably had reference to the ordinary transport wagons used on this occasion for conveying sick and wounded.

During the 1864 Convention in Geneva, an agreement was made by several European countries to recognize the neutrality of hospitals, the sick and wounded, and all persons connected with relief service, as well as to adopt a protective sign or badge.

In America, a similar organization was functioning during the Civil War. Clara Barton and a circle of acquaintances founded the American Red Cross in Washington, D.C. on May 21, 1881. Barton first heard of the Swiss-inspired international Red Cross network while visiting Europe following the Civil War. Returning home, she campaigned for an American Red Cross society and for ratification of the Geneva Convention protecting the war-injured, which the United States ratified in 1882.[3]

As we know, most ambulance innovations took place during wartime, which were then adapted to civilian life. American hospitals initiated their own ambulance service during the late 1860s. Horse-drawn, these ambulance services had a movable floor that could be drawn out to receive the

---

3   A brief history of the American Red Cross. Available at: www.redcross.org. Accessed August 17, 2010.

patient. Beneath the driver's seat was a container with a quart of brandy, two tourniquets, six bandages, six small sponges, splint material, blankets, and a 2-ounce vial of persulphate of iron (used as an astringent). This was considered the early day trauma bag. With the arrival of the automobile came a different type of ambulance, first appearing in 1899. During World War I, many ambulances were adapted from buses and taxis. In 1867, Major General Rucker won the "best of kind" for an ambulance that was adopted as the regulation ambulance. It had extra springs on the floor, more elasticity to the stretchers, and improved ventilation.

In 1937, the world's oldest builder of ambulances Hess & Eisenhardt Company from Cincinnati, Ohio, sold the first air-conditioned ambulance built in America. Developed with the idea that the ambulance should be a prehospital emergency room, these precursors of the modern ambulance were filled with medicine cabinets, roof lights, and two-way radios.

Moving right along, emergency medical services (EMS) personnel really should understand the history of how "modern EMS" evolved. Although the history of EMS won't get you through cardiology emergency or trauma, it will definitely make you respect what our predecessors did prior to Kendrick extrication devices, IVs, epinephrine, and oh yeah, 12-leads, capnography, and cardiopulmonary resuscitation (CPR).

In 1865, the first hospital-based ambulance service in the United States was created in Cincinnati, Ohio, which was based out of Commercial Hospital. This hospital is now called Cincinnati General Hospital, and EMS is operated by the fire department. Other services soon followed: Grady Hospital in Atlanta, Charity Hospital in New Orleans, and several hospitals in New York City and other major cities. (In December 1869, the first month of operation, the ambulance service of the Free Hospital of New York [Bellevue] ran 74 calls. By 1870, a total of 1466 ambulance calls were run.) The dispatch system was much different from that used today. The hospital rang a bell, which triggered a weight to fall, lighting the gas lamp to wake the physician and the driver. It also caused the harness, saddle, and collar to drop on the horse while opening the stable doors; however, this alarm system was modern for its time and was limited to large cities.[4]

Ambulance service was not confined to ground units. During the Civil War, train ambulances and steam boat hospitals were used, and street car/trolley ambulances were popular in some cities in the late 1800s.

The medevac helicopter, now commonplace, first came into service as a means of evacuating combat patients in Korea and Vietnam. Now medevacs

---

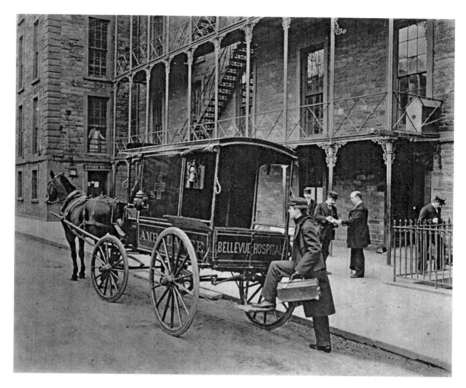

FIGURE I-2. Photo of an ambulance in New York City in 1895. *(From The Byron Collection, Museum of the City of New York, New York, New York.)*

are an invaluable resource during long-distance transports of critically ill or injured patients.

Forty years ago, you couldn't stand up in an ambulance. And the term "ambulance" had somewhat of a fluid definition, as equipment and personnel training differed from one area of the United States to another. Whereas modern-day EMS came about as a result of a 1966 publication by the National Academy of Sciences, paramedic-level care was the result of concerns over coronary care.

In the late 1960s, coronary artery disease was the country's number one cause of death, claiming approximately 400,000 lives per year. Roughly 70% of those deaths occurred in the prehospital setting. It is interesting to note that it is still the number one cause of death in the United States 50 years later (according to the Centers for Disease Control and Prevention). Physicians across the nation, from Pittsburgh and Columbus to Seattle

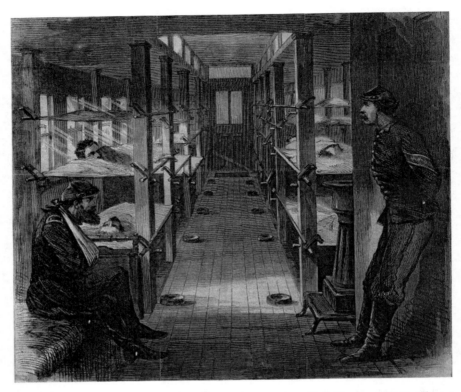

FIGURE I-3. Depiction of a hospital train from the American Civil War era. *(Sketched by Theodore R. Davis. Originally published in Harper's Weekly, February 27, 1864.)*

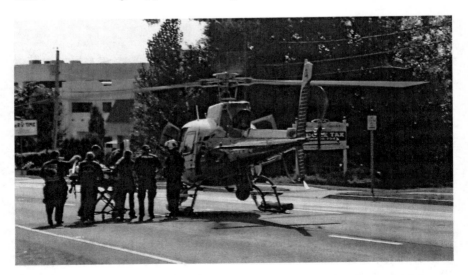

FIGURE I-4. The medevac helicopter. *(Used with permission from Peter A. DiPrima, Jr.)*

and Los Angeles, recognized that lives could be saved using a prehospital medical care system. However, those administering advanced cardiac care would have to be highly trained and have the ability to mobilize within minutes.

Luckily, programs in Europe had been established and reported on. Physicians in the United States used Dr. Pantridge's work from Belfast and similar programs in Moscow as starting points. American doctors, however, found that the European model of physician-staffed ambulances didn't suit the American landscape. By 1970, numerous programs had been instituted to train non-physicians to provide advanced medical care. These new healthcare professionals would become known as "paramedics."

Let's not forget Hollywood's *Emergency!* This TV show originally aired on NBC between 1972 and 1977. The show centered on Station 51 and Rampart Emergency Hospital. Station 51 housed a squad and an engine (the station has had both a Crown and a Ward LaFrance) with a normal crew of six, two of which were paramedics. The show began with the pilot movie showing the paramedic program in its infancy, before legislation was in effect to allow the paramedics to function independently. It follows the characters of paramedics John Gage and Roy DeSoto to the point when they are promoted to captain. Most episodes were split between rescue scenes in the "field" and follow-up treatment at the hospital afterward. As corny as it may seem compared with today's standards, the television program educated the common folk about what EMS and paramedics are capable of and the show opened the door to today's paramedic.[5]

FEDERAL LEGISLATION, 1966–1980: THE BIRTH OF MODERN-DAY EMS

Modern EMS came about in 1966 as a result of heavy involvement of the federal government and a monumental publication. The National Academy of Sciences' National Research Council produced a 37-page paper entitled "Accidental Death and Disability: The Neglected Diseases of Modern Society," commonly referred to as the "White Paper."[6]

---

5 Yokley R, Sutherland R. *Emergency! Behind the Scene.* Sudbury, MA: Jones and Bartlett Publishers; 2007.
6 National Academy of Sciences. Accidental Death and Disability: The Neglected Disease of Modern Society. White Paper. 1966.

▓ Looking back at how it all started...

Between 1963 and 1966, The National Academy of Sciences instructed its Committees on Trauma, Shock, and Anesthesia, along with special task forces of the Division of Medical Services, to comprehensively review the status of EMS accessible to accident victims. The committees reviewed everything to do with emergency care at the time, from ambulance services and communication systems to emergency departments and intensive care facilities.[7]

Once done, the National Research Council reported that in 1965, 52 million accidental injuries occurred in the United States, killing 107,000 and disabling over 10 million. The Council went on to report numerous factors that would require early and timely intervention, including the following:

1. The general public is insensitive to the magnitude of the problem of accidental death and injury.
2. Millions lack instruction in basic first aid.
3. Few are adequately trained in the advanced techniques of CPR, childbirth, or other lifesaving measures, yet every ambulance and rescue squad attendant, policeman, firefighter, paramedic worker, and worker in high-risk industries should be trained.
4. Local political authorities have neglected their responsibility to provide optimal EMS.
5. Research on trauma has not been supported or identified by the National Institutes of Health on a level consistent with its importance as the fourth leading cause of death and the primary cause of disability.
6. Potentials of the U.S. Public Health Service programs in accident prevention and EMS have not been fully exploited.
7. Data are lacking on which to determine the number of individuals whose lives are lost or injuries are compounded by misguided attempts at rescue or first aid, absence of physicians at the scene of injury, unsuitable ambulances with inadequate equipment and untrained attendants, lack of traffic control, or the lack of voice communication facilities.
8. Helicopter ambulances have not been adapted to civilian peacetime needs.
9. Emergency departments of hospitals are overcrowded, some are archaic, and there are no systematic surveys on which to base requirements for space, equipment, or staffing for present, let alone future, needs.

---

7 A Historical Overview of EMS System Development in the US: 1960s and 1970s. Available at: www.semp.US. Accessed September 22, 2010.

10. Fundamental research in shock and trauma is inadequately supported.

11. Medical and health-related organizations have failed to join forces to apply knowledge already available to advance the treatment of trauma or to educate the public and inform the U.S. Congress.

In 1960, the President's Commission on Highway Safety was formed and issued its report "Health, Medical Care, and Transportation of the Injured." The report focused solely on the growing problem of highway-related accidental injury and "...established 18 standards for improving highway safety."

The U.S. Congress responded quickly to these reports. The National Highway Safety Act of 1966 (P.L. 89-564, 80 Stat. 731) would provide $48 million between 1966 and 1973 through the Department of Transportation. Additionally, federal programs through the Department of Health, Education, and Welfare, as well as the Division of Emergency Medical Services, would provide over $73 million for various EMS projects.[8]

In November of 1973, after overriding a presidential veto of the bill, federal funding for EMS was expanded with the passage of the Emergency Medical Services Systems Act of 1973 (P.L. 93-154). The EMS Systems Act authorized the Department of Health, Education, and Welfare to award Regional Medical Program (RMP) grants for:

1. The establishment and initial operation of EMS systems.

2. Projects for the expansion and improvement of EMS systems.

3. Support of research in emergency medical techniques, methods, devices, and delivery.

The EMS Systems Act authorized funds of $30 million for 1974, $60 million for 1975, and $70 million for 1976.[9] The act also stipulated that an Interagency Committee on Emergency Medical Services be established in order to fully evaluate the sufficiency of governmental activities. An EMS system could be several counties in size and would be managed by a single public or nonprofit agency. In addition, 15 components of an EMS system were defined:

1. Manpower

2. Training

---

8   U.S. Department of Transportation, National Highway Safety Bureau. 1969. Report on Activities under the Highway Safety Act. Washington, DC: The Bureau; 1969.

9   National Highway Safety Administration, Federal Highway Administration, U.S. Department of Transportation. Uniform Procedures for State Highway Safety Programs. Available at: www. Nhtsa. dot.gov. Accessed July 2, 2010.

3. Communications

4. Transportation

5. Facilities

6. Critical care units

7. Public safety agencies

8. Community participation

9. Accessibility to care

10. Transfer of patients

11. Standardized patient record-keeping

12. Public information and education

13. Disaster planning

14. Mutual aid agreements

15. Review and evaluation

The Health Services Administration of the Department of Health, Education, and Welfare also provided funds for the planning and expansion of EMS systems. Between 1974 and 1975, over 200 grants were awarded through this legislation. Initial funding provided by the EMS Systems Act of 1973 ended in 1976. Legislation was then immediately introduced to amend and extend the federal funding. In response to the proposed extension of the act, the General Accounting Office and the Comptroller General of the United States issued a report in June of 1975 to the U.S. Congress. This report reviewed the EMS system program and stated that "...although the progress is being made in the development of regional systems, the continued viability of such systems is not assured when Federal funding terminates."

Therefore, in October 1976, the EMS Systems Act of 1973 was revised and amended as Public Law 94-573. The extended act authorized "...the appropriation of specified sums for purposes of making EMS grants and contracts in fiscal years 1976 through 1979." These amendments later led, in 1978, to the creation of 304 EMS regions in the United States.

In 1978, the National Academy of Sciences' Committee of Emergency Medical Services published a paper entitled "Emergency Medical Services at Midpassage." As a retrospective review of advancements made in EMS over the preceding 12 years, the paper stated that "the availability of developmental funds ... has resulted in significant improvement in many communities." However, though highlighting the improvement in prehospital care, the paper also called attention to the possibility of federal funding coming to a sudden end.

By 1979, it was apparent that the majority of EMS systems established and sustained with federal grants were failing to plan for self-sufficiency. One provision of the 1976 amended EMS Systems Act was that EMS systems across the nation must plan their own financial futures. This meant that systems receiving large amounts of federal funds now had to seek financial commitments from local governments or nonprofit agencies in order to maintain their regional operations. Because of the careless nature of the majority of EMS systems across the country, large amounts of money would have to be secured in a very short period of time, because federal assistance would soon come to an abrupt end in the 1980s.

EARLY ADVOCACY

While senators were battling in Washington, D.C., James O. Page was paving his own road of prehospital advocacy and advancement. The former Los

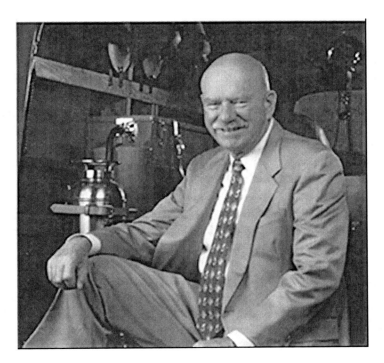

FIGURE I-5. Photograph of James O. Page. *(Reproduced with permission from: Never forgotten: remembering EMS leader James O. Page. Journal of Emergency Medical Services [JEMS] web site, http://www.jems.com. Published August 30, 2009. Accessed January 17, 2012.)*

Angeles County Battalion Chief had already helped set up North Carolina's statewide EMS system and was now established in Buffalo, New York, managing a federally funded EMS project encompassing an eight-county area of western New York. Using his resources to their full potential, Page prepared the first national paramedic survey.

Questionnaires were sent to EMS directors and personnel in all 50 states. Within 5 months, every state had been accounted for and data analysis had begun. Results showed that, by 1975, paramedics were operational in 46 states.

Based on Page's research, and using funds from the Lakes Area Regional Medical Programs, "The National Study of Paramedic Law and Policy" was published. The report stated that "... more than half the paramedic programs then in existence had begun without clear-cut authorizing legislation from their respective state legislatures." And, between 1969 and 1976, paramedic services had been established without legal authority in 25 states. Also disclosed within Page's report was that no less than 15 different titles were being used throughout the country when referring to paramedics. This led the newly formed National Association of EMTs, in 1976, to adopt an official name for advanced-level prehospital medical providers, emergency medical technician–paramedic, or EMT-P.

The report garnered national notice. After being distributed to over 150,000 healthcare workers, within 2 years, only two states were still without paramedic legislation. Page also teamed up with the Department of Transportation to create the Model State Emergency Medical Services Statute.

Also published in 1976, a national survey of paramedics dug a little deeper than Page's. The survey distributed by Dr. Elliott Salenger, medical director of the Emergency Medical Services Division of Los Angeles County's Department of Health, and Joe Slotkin, student at the University of California at Los Angeles, made an effort to geographically locate every paramedic service in the country. They found that 214 paramedic services were operational in the United States. Because of the fluid definition of "paramedic" at the time, the results of the study were deemed inconclusive.

As data were being received and analyzed for the Page and Salenger-Slotkin studies, the Department of Transportation named the University of Pittsburgh's Department of Anesthesia and Critical Care Medicine as the recipient of the federal contract to develop the first national paramedic training course. As chairman of the university's department, Dr. Peter Safar would delegate responsibility to Dr. Nancy Caroline, former medical director for Pittsburgh's Freedom House paramedics.

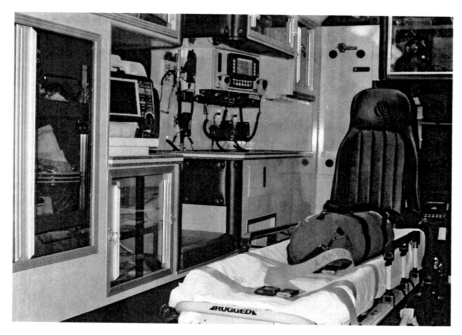

FIGURE I-6. Photo of a modern-day ambulance. *(Used with permission from Peter A. DiPrima, Jr.)*

Dr. Caroline surveyed 30 paramedic programs across the country and soon found enormous discrepancies. She found that training programs ranged from 100 to 1200 hours in length and either covered medical and trauma topics comprehensively or focused solely on cardiac care. Dr. Caroline also found large inconsistencies regarding training in patient assessment and medical terminology. Although a few training programs covered these topics fully, most paid little to no attention to them. Additionally, whereas arrhythmia recognition/therapy and intravenous fluid therapy were nearly complete in coverage, respiratory emergencies were included in only one-third of paramedic programs.

Today's ambulances are now literally emergency rooms on wheels and come equipped with some amazing new technology. Lifesaving equipment such as defibrillators and monitors that can transmit a complete 12-lead electrocardiograph (ECG) directly to the emergency department, as well as advanced airways, drugs, and intravenous therapy to the latest handheld computers are just some of the innovative equipment and training the modern paramedic utilizes. The advancement of the ambulance has definitely come a long way from early battlefield times. As technology advances, we will continue to see changes in the equipment that is carried, but the framework that is recognizable today will be here to stay for time to come.

Please take the time to recognize some of our modern EMS leaders who have passed away.

James O. Page, August 7, 1936–September 4, 2004

Dr. Nancy Lee Caroline, June 27, 1944–December 12, 2002

Dr. Peter Safar, April 12, 1924–August 2, 2003

CHAPTER 2

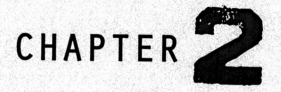

YOUR ROLE IN THE HEALTHCARE SYSTEM AS AN EMS PROVIDER

As a paramedic, we have to be a multifaceted, independent healthcare provider that provides emergency care and at times performs as a psychologist, sociologist, mediator, respiratory therapist, interventionist, and whatever else comes along at the scene of an emergency. So what are our current roles and responsibilities as a paramedic? Excerpt from the Department of Transportation:

National Highway Traffic Safety Administration (NHTSA) as defined in the 1998 Paramedic Curriculum; the Paramedic must be a confident leader who can accept the challenge and high degree of responsibility entailed in the position. The Paramedic must have excellent judgment and be able to prioritize decisions and act quickly in the best interest of the patient, must be self-disciplined, able to develop patient rapport, interview hostile patients, maintain safe distance, and recognize and utilize communication unique to diverse multicultural groups and ages within those groups. The Paramedic must be able to function independently at optimum level in a non-structured environment that is constantly changing. Even though the Paramedic is generally part of a two-person team often working with a lower skill and knowledge level Basic EMT, it is the Paramedic who is held responsible for safe and therapeutic administration of drugs (including narcotics). Therefore, the Paramedic must not only be knowledgeable about medications, but must be able to apply this knowledge in a practical sense. Knowledge and practical application of medications include thoroughly knowing and understanding the general properties of all types of drugs including analgesics, anesthetics, anti-anxiety drugs, sedatives and hypnotics, anti-convulsants, central nervous system stimulants, psychotherapeutics(which include antidepressants and other anti-psychotics), anti-cholinergics, cholinergics, muscle relaxants, anti-dysrhythmics, anti-hypertensives, anticoagulants, diuretics, bronchodilators, opthalmics, pituitary drugs, gastrointestinal drugs, hormones, antibiotics, anti-fungals, anti-inflammatories, serums, vaccines, anti-parasitics, and others.

The Paramedic is personally responsible, legally, ethically, and morally for each drug administered, for using correct precautions and techniques, observing and documenting the effects of the drugs administered, keeping one's own pharmacological knowledgebase current as to changes and trends in administration and use, keeping abreast of all contraindications to administration of specific drugs to patients based on their constitutional make-up, and using drug reference literature.

The responsibility of the Paramedic includes obtaining a comprehensive drug history from the patient that includes names of drugs, strength, daily usage and dosage. The Paramedic must take into consideration that many factors, in relation to the history given, can affect the type of medication to be given. For example, some patients may be taking several medications prescribed by several different doctors and some may lose track of what they have or have not taken. Some may be using non-prescription/over-the counter drugs. Awareness of drug reactions and the synergistic effects of drugs combined with other medicines and in some instances, food, are imperative. The Paramedic must also take into consideration the possible risks of medication administered to a pregnant mother and the fetus, keeping in mind that drug may cross the placenta.

The Paramedic must be cognizant of the impact of medications on pediatric patients based on size and weight. The Paramedic must also be aware of the special concerns related to newborn and geriatric patients and the physiological effects of aging such as the way newborns breathe or how easily skin can tear in the geriatric population. There must be an awareness of the high abuse potential of controlled substances and the potential for addiction; therefore, the Paramedic must be thorough in report writing and able to justify why a particular narcotic was used and why a particular amount was given. The ability to measure and re-measure drip rates for controlled substances/medications are essential. Once medication is stopped or not used, the Paramedic must send back unused portions to the proper inventory arena.

The Paramedic must be able to apply basic principles of mathematics to the calculation of problems associated with medication dosages, perform conversion problems, and differentiate temperature readings between centigrade and Fahrenheit scales. The Paramedic must be able to use proper advanced life support equipment and supplies (i.e. proper size of intravenous needles) based on patient's age and condition of veins, and be able to locate sites for obtaining blood samples and perform this task.

Paramedics must also be able to administer medication intravenously, by gastric tube, orally and rectally, and comply with universal precautions and body substance isolation, including disposing of contaminated items and equipment properly.

The Paramedic must be able to apply knowledge and skills to assist overdosed patients through antidotes, and have knowledge of poisons and be able to administer treatment. The Paramedic must be knowledgeable as to the stages drugs/medications go through once they have entered the patient's system and be cognizant that route of administration is critical in relation to patient's needs and the effect that occurs. The Paramedic must also be capable of providing advanced life support emergency medical procedures to patients including conducting of and interpreting electrocardiograms (EKGs), electrical interventions to support cardiac function, endotracheal intubations (in airway management), relief of pneumothorax and administration of appropriate intravenous fluids and drugs under direction of an off-site designated physician.

The Paramedic is a person who must not only remain calm while working in difficult and stressful circumstances, but must be capable of staying focused while assuming the leadership role inherent in carrying out the functions of the position. Good judgment along with advanced knowledge and technical skills are essential in directing other team members to assist as needed.

The Paramedic must be able to provide top quality care, concurrently handle high levels of stress, and be willing to take on the personal responsibility required of the position. This includes not only all legal ramifications for precise documentation, but also the responsibility for using the knowledge and skills acquired in real, life-threatening emergency situations.

The Paramedic must be able to deal with adverse and often dangerous situations which include responding to calls in districts known to have high crime and mortality rates.

Self-confidence is critical, as is a desire to work with people, solid emotional stability, tolerance for high stress, and the ability to meet the physical, intellectual, and cognitive requirements demanded by this position.[1]

THE ROLES AND RESPONSIBILITIES OF A PARAMEDIC

The roles and responsibilities of the paramedic are increasingly changing throughout the United States. Today, the U.S. healthcare system is underfunded and plagued by limited supplies and increasing demand for services. Emergency medical services (EMS) is often touted as a "public health safety net," a service to which the public can turn when no other option is available for immediate healthcare needs. Similarly, hospital emergency departments are increasingly called upon to provide primary care services for the growing portion of the public without adequate health insurance or primary care resources. At the same time, changes in health technology and reimbursement have led to decreased hospital lengths of stay and earlier discharge of patients. As a result, patients may be sent home while still at risk for postsurgical or postevent (medical) complications. In addition, patients are being sent home with technology that has, until now, been seen primarily in the hospital. Examples include medication infusion devices such as IV pumps, patient-controlled anesthesia (PCA) devices, ventilators, and continuous positive airway pressure (CPAP) devices, and left ventricular assist devices (LVADs), to mention a few. When complications arise, patients access the EMS system and are transported to the emergency department (ED). This has added a higher volume of critically ill patients for EMS and a new subset of patients with special needs and considerations. As both the EMS system and EDs struggle to fulfill these roles, it is important to note that neither was designed with these roles in mind. The result has been chronic overcrowding of EDs, long wait times, and ED diversions.

---

1   U.S. Department of Transportation, National Highway Traffic Safety Administration. Paramedic National Curriculum.

Excerpt from the Department of Transportation:

Aptitudes required for work of this nature are good physical stamina, endurance, and body condition that would not be adversely affected by frequently having to walk, stand, lift, carry, and balance at times, in excess of 125 pounds. Motor coordination is necessary because over uneven terrain, the patient's, the Paramedic's, and other workers' well-being must not be jeopardized.

The Paramedic provides the most extensive pre-hospital care and may work for fire departments, private ambulance services, police departments or hospitals. Response times for nature of work are dependent upon nature of call. For example, a Paramedic working for a private ambulance service that transports the elderly from nursing homes to routine medical appointments and check-ups may endure somewhat less stressful circumstances than the Paramedic who works primarily with 911 calls in a district known to have high crime rates. Thus, the particular stresses inherent in the role of the Paramedic can vary, depending on place and type of employment.

However, in general, in the analyst's opinion, the Paramedic must be flexible to meet the demands of the ever-changing emergency scene. When emergencies exist, the situation can be complex and care of the patient must be started immediately. In essence, the Paramedic in the EMS system uses advanced training and equipment to extend emergency physician services to the ambulance. The Paramedic must be able to make accurate independent judgments while following oral directives. The ability to perform duties in a timely manner is essential, as it could mean the difference between life and death for the patient.

Use of the telephone or radio dispatch for coordination of prompt emergency services is required, as is a pager, depending on place of employment. Accurately discerning street names through map reading, and correctly distinguishing house numbers or business addresses are essential to task completion in the most expedient manner. Concise and accurate verbal description of a patient's condition is a critical skill for paramedic to acquire. The Paramedic must also be able to accurately report, orally and in writing all relevant patient data. At times, reporting may require a detailed narrative on extenuating circumstances or conditions that go beyond what is required on a prescribed form. In some instances, the Paramedic must enter data on computer. Verbal skills and reasoning skills are used extensively.[2]

---

2   U.S. Department of Transportation, National Highway Traffic Safety Administration. Paramedic National Curriculum.

You should have a basic understanding of what your roles and responsibilities are fresh out of medic school. The reality is that where you are working or volunteering will determine what level and to what extreme you will be utilizing your basic paramedic-level training. Starting my career as a volunteer emergency medical technician (EMT) on Long Island was definitely different from working as an EMT and paramedic in New York City. I worked in some of the toughest neighborhoods in the Unites States. IV skills, patient history taking, and medication administration are the same, but operationally, geographically, and sheer call volume, well, it was definitely different! I've been in EMS for 23 years and have seen incredible changes and progress from the late 1980s until now. One of the largest (and most unexpected) is the sense of professionalism and acceptance that the traditional medical community has granted (and we've earned). I'm sure most old-timers out there can remember the days of being treated very poorly by registered nurses (RNs) and mostly ignored by the ED docs. Those days are long gone. Advanced treatment in many areas of the country is expected. So what's in our future? Each state has the statutory authority and responsibility to regulate EMS within its borders. This makes things somewhat difficult. Currently, we do not have a national standard of care, so care varies from state to state, county to county, and sometimes town to town. EMS personnel are unique healthcare professionals because they provide medical care and transportation in an out-of-hospital setting with medical oversight (our system or agency medical director, protocols, and medical control). It's important to remember that EMS personnel are not independent practitioners. This is why we treat with a series of protocols that are defined by standing orders or through contact with a physician (on- or off-line medical direction). Although the "practice" is not independent, it is relatively unsupervised and often has little backup. Therefore, EMS personnel must be able to exercise considerable judgment (common sense) and problem-solving and decision-making skills. Most EMS personnel work in emergency medical organizations that respond to emergency calls. Emergency response is typically a local government function (or is contracted by local government to a private entity). In most communities, citizens call 911 when they need emergency medical care, and the appropriate EMS resources are dispatched. EMS personnel respond and provide care to the patient in the setting in which the patient became ill or injured, including the home, field, work, industrial, and recreational settings. In the case of emergency calls, EMS personnel are unique in that they typically have a duty to act.

Taking It to the Streets

I remember my very first call as a paramedic. A BLS crew was calling for medics for a patient in acute pulmonary edema. My partner and I arrive, enter the apartment, and the lead EMT says, "Good, the medics are here!" I turned around and looked behind me, forgetting I was the medic!

In some areas of the country, waiting to be triaged in the ED can take in excess of 10 minutes, which could be a real nail biter when you are applying positive-pressure ventilation to a patient with a bag valve mask (BVM). Obviously, these ridiculously busy EDs are overburdened, understaffed, and definitely underpaid. I can recall a conversation with an ED nurse who was at her wits end being pulled in 15 directions. Well, let's say she took all her frustration out on me and my partner and in front of our patient. Needless to say, that type of behavior doesn't give patients a warm and fuzzy feeling when they don't feel well and they don't feel welcome. Minus her expletives, she said, "Don't you see how busy we are! Why did you bring us another one?" My only answer to her was, "If you're busy, we're busy! Who do you think brought those patients here? Obviously, EMS!"

NHTSA: IMPLEMENTATION GUIDE

Excerpt: EMS Agenda for the Future "The Vision"

Our nation's health care system is in flux. Efforts to reduce cost and improve the effectiveness of health care are leading to fundamental changes in the way the public accesses—and pays for—medical treatment. Recognizing the skills and strengths of pre-hospital professionals and the importance of superior EMS care, the National Highway Traffic Safety Administration and the Health Resources and Services Administration joined with leaders from the EMS community in 1996 to create a strategic plan for building the next millennium's EMS system.

The EMS Agenda for the Future envisions EMS as the linchpin joining today's isolated public safety, health care and public health systems. While emergency response must remain our foundation, EMS of tomorrow will be a community-based health management system that provides surveillance, identification, intervention and evaluation of injury and disease. This role strengthens the essential value of EMS as the community's emergency medical safety net.

Emergency medical services (EMS) of the future will be community-based health management that is fully integrated with the overall health care system. It will have the ability to identify and modify illness and injury risks, provide acute illness and injury care and follow-up, and contribute to treatment of chronic conditions and community health monitoring. This new entity will be developed from redistribution of existing health care resources and will be integrated with other health care providers and public health and public safety agencies. It will improve community health and result in more appropriate use of acute health care resources. EMS will remain the public's emergency medical safety net.[3]

Ricardo Martinez, MD
Administrator
National Highway Traffic Safety Administration

As with anything that involves medicine, there are many legal and legislative changes that need to occur in order for EMS to mature into this licensed entity. There is a very strong drive to produce a national model that revolves around the following areas:

- National EMS core content
- National EMS scope of practice model
- National EMS education standards
- National EMS education program accreditation
- National EMS certification

To guarantee the best EMS system in the future, we need to improve our foundation!

SO WHAT EXACTLY ARE OUR ROLES AND RESPONSIBILITIES ANYWAY?

Take a deep breath. You learned a lot, but you don't know what you don't know. The most important part of making the transition from BLS Provider to Paramedic is becoming a leader, and a good listener— a *medical detective* so to speak.

---

3 EMS Agenda for the Future, Implementation Guide. Available at: www.nhtsa.gov. Accessed September 21, 2010.

Dress the part. Shine your boots, press your uniform, and tuck in your shirt. First impressions speak volumes. Mere presence and presentation is a display of leadership, illustrating control. The emergency is over when the paramedics arrive on scene.

Be respectful to your patient and crew members. If you treat them as if you would your own family, you can never go wrong. Look, listen, and feel. Not only part of your patient assessment, but be fully aware of your surroundings. Look for hazards, access, and egress. Note living conditions, lighting, heat, cold, stairs, children, pets, rodents? What odors or malodors? Prescription bottles, medical supplies, family, and bystanders? Alcohol, food, or lack thereof? Ask a lot of questions, before you start your treatment. Don't create a sketch; paint a picture. Be thorough. Once you arrive at a presumptive diagnosis, ask more questions. Listen. Don't feel obligated to act quickly—more important to act accurately. Keep listening. Keep learning.

Christopher VanHouten, NREMT-P

FOUR RESPONSIBILITIES TO REMEMBER

▨ I. Respect (R-E-S-P-E-C-T)

Paramedics must respond with respect, to both the physical and the emotional needs of patients. This means putting aside personal beliefs and prejudices. They must also be respectful of patient confidentiality, just as any other health professional must be. "Into whatever homes I enter, I will go into them for the benefit of only the sick and injured, never revealing what I see or hear in the lives of men unless required by law," states the EMT Oath, written by Dr. Charles B. Gillespie, and adopted by the National Association of Emergency Medical Technicians.

Respect has great importance in everyday life. As children, we are taught (one hopes) to respect our parents, teachers, and elders. As a fundamental professional value, respect should permeate a paramedic's relationship with his or her patients. Outwardly, respect is manifested by behaviors that reinforce a patient's dignity: simply introducing ourselves and explaining our roles carefully; addressing patients as Mr. or Ms., rather than using first names; asking permission before examining patients; sitting and making eye contact; paying close attention when patients speak to us. These are all well-understood ways to convey respect. Unintrusiveness is less often emphasized as an aspect of respectfulness. Patients give paramedics unrivaled access to their privacy. This vulnerability of patients must be counterbalanced by respect. Thus, we should expose as little as possible when examining private parts of patients and be extremely respectful of confidentiality. We should avoid discussing patients with anyone not involved in their care and certainly never mention patients in public places.

2. Skills Mastery

Like other medical professionals, paramedics take an oath to do no harm. Paramedics may face legal liability for failing to perform their jobs appropriately. However, they also have an ethical responsibility to make sure they have a mastery of the skills needed to do the job effectively. This means participating in continuing education and refresher trainings. Innovations are constantly changing the medical field. As a result, paramedics must make sure that they have a good working knowledge of new concepts and modalities in emergency patient care. Additionally, they should review their own performance on a constant basis as a way to ensure that they are always improving the level of service they provide.

3. Cooperation

Paramedics must report with honesty anything they believe can help a patient's health. They must also work harmoniously with other emergency medical personnel, including doctors and nurses, to ensure a patient's health is the top priority. In instances where they are responding to situations alongside other emergency responders, such as firefighters and police, paramedics have an ethical responsibility to be cooperative and respectful of other emergency efforts occurring simultaneously with their own.

4. Patient Advocacy

Paramedics should work with citizens and other healthcare professionals to promote a high standard of medical care for all, according to the EMT Code of Ethics. They should also "demonstrate concern for the competence of other members of the Emergency Medical Services healthcare team."

Our roles and responsibilities will continue to change, as will medicine. The landscape of medicine is significantly changing because of financial constraints choking the U.S. healthcare system. This in turn will further expand the future paramedic's roles, becoming involved in not only emergency medicine, but also primary and long-term care. Our older population—defined as persons 65 years or older—numbered 39.6 million in 2009 (the latest year for which data are available). Baby Boomers represented 12.9%

of the U.S. population, about one in every eight Americans. According to the Department of Health and Human Services, by 2030, there will be about 72.1 million older persons, more than twice their number in 2000. People 65+ represented 12.4% of the population in the year 2000 but are expected to grow to be 19% of the population by 2030. Guess who is going to be filling this large healthcare gap? Yep, you guessed right: Paramedics.

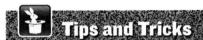
Tips and Tricks

True professionals establish excellence as their goal and never allow themselves to become complacent about their performance.

CHAPTER 3

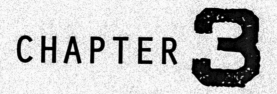

CAREER OPPORTUNITIES IN EMS: NOW YOU'RE A PARAMEDIC!

So what's next? After graduation, the next step is to decide where and for whom you want to work. Because of the dynamic nature of individual state regulations, providing intricate information on how to be certified or licensed in each state is next to impossible. Appendix A lists contact information for each state, along with its website. It will guide you in the process as outlined by each entity when it comes to reciprocity, certification, and licensure.

CERTIFICATION VERSUS LICENSURE

Summarized from the National Association of Emergency Medical Technicians:

Although some EMS agencies continue to use the terms certification and licensure interchangeably, there are important functional distinctions between the two. The federal government has defined "certification" as the process by which a nongovernmental organization grants recognition to an individual who has met predetermined qualifications specified by that organization. Similarly, the National Commission for Certifying Agencies has recently defined certification as "a process, often voluntary, by which individuals who have demonstrated the level of knowledge and skill required in the profession, occupation, role, or skill are identified to the public and other stakeholders."

There are three hallmarks of certification; certification is

1. a voluntary process.
2. by a private organization.
3. for the purpose of providing the public information on those individuals who have successfully completed the certification process (usually entailing successful completion of educational and testing requirements) and demonstrated their ability to perform their profession competently.

Nearly every medical profession certifies its members in some way. Private certifying boards certify physician specialists. Although certification may assist a physician in obtaining hospital privileges or participating as a preferred provider within a health insurer's network, it does not affect his or her legal authority to practice medicine. Licensure, on the other hand, is the state's grant of legal authority, pursuant to the state's police powers, to practice a profession within a designated scope of practice. Under the licensure system, states define, by statute, the tasks and function or scope of practice of a profession and provide that these tasks may be legally performed only by those who are licensed. As such, licensure prohibits anyone who is not licensed from practicing the profession, regardless of whether the individual has been certified by a private organization. For example, a surgeon can practice medicine in any state in which he or she is licensed regardless of certification by the American Board of Surgery. Confusion between the terms "certification" and "licensure" arises because many states call their licensure processes "certification," particularly when they incorporate the standards and requirements of private certifying bodies in their licensing statutes and require that an individual be certified in order to have state authorization to practice. For example, the use of "certification" by the National Registry of Emergency Medical Technicians by some states as a basis for granting individuals the right to practice as EMTs and calling the authorization granted "certification" is an example of this practice.

Regardless of what descriptive title is used by a state agency, if an occupation has a defined statutory or regulatory scope of practice and only individuals authorized by the state can perform those functions and activities, the authorized individuals are licensed. It does not matter if the authorization is called something other than a license; the authorization has the legal effect of a license. The various state offices of EMS or like agencies serve as the state licensing agencies.

CAREER PATH

When you started EMS, you might have thought this would be a good way to give back to the community or make some extra money; however, over the last year, you have been seriously considering a career in EMS. I mean, what the heck, you just finished paramedic school. As you look through your training history, it becomes apparent that in order to make a career out of EMS, you need to take some very important steps. What courses do you take first? What direction would you like your career to take? What path is the most appropriate for you?

The good news is that at any time during your EMS career, you can change the focus of your studies without having to take steps backward. For example, if you start out being a career paramedic and want to get into EMS management, a few classes can help you achieve that goal. The reverse is also true.

The following five tips may help you choose or switch your current career path:

1. **Continue your education**—I can't say enough about furthering your education. The more credentials, classes, and continuing medical education credits you earn, the more marketable you will be. When going to national or state conferences, choose tracks that best fit with your overall career goals. If you are currently an EMT and think you might be interested in becoming a paramedic, take a few of the courses listed in the Advanced Life Support (ALS) track. Likewise, most EMS conferences now feature management courses; expand your knowledge by attending one of these. In addition to conferences, seek out EMS courses that offer college credit, certificates, or degrees.

2. **Plan your career**—Take time to plan your career. Goal-setting is a skill that takes time to develop. Whether you choose the operations route, management, or even being an EMS educator, you need to set goals for yourself. Start with small, attainable goals like completing a paramedic course or completing an associate's degree in business management. Your small goals should add up and feed into your big-picture goal. Preplanning will help steer the direction of your education and provide milestones and checkpoints for your professional achievements.

3. **Be flexible**—Keep an open mind to changes in your goal-setting process. Know when to push through and when to reevaluate your situation. There really are no hard and fast rules about when to evaluate how well your process is going; however, as discussed in the last section, you will reach milestones throughout your path. At those times, it is a good idea to take a step back and look at how well your plan is working. Don't be afraid to change direction. There are many opportunities from operations (EMT/paramedic/line supervisor) to management (training/middle management/human resources/billing) that you may have not considered.

4. **Try different organizations**—Within the scope of paramedicine, individual organizations perform general EMS functions differently. Agencies have different policies and procedures that differentiate them. Try commercial EMS agencies and volunteer or mixed organizations to gain as much knowledge in operations as possible. This will become particularly important if your career path steers you toward management.

5. **Find a mentor**—Mentors are an important part of career success. We don't put enough emphasis on finding people to guide us through our careers. A seasoned paramedic can provide a world of guidance to a new EMT. Similarly, an experienced EMS manager can assist newer supervisors in gaining necessary skills. How do you know what you are getting into? Trying to navigate EMS systems can be intimidating, even for personnel who have been around for a while. Imagine what it's like to be starting out in a new system. Mentors will not only teach you how to take a blood pressure correctly, they will show you why you are taking a specific action. When you hit a crossroad between management and operations career paths, a mentor can help you ask the right questions to make a wise decision.

Your career will take many turns over time, and there will be plenty of opportunities if you position yourself along the way. Two important things to remember about planning your career: It is never too late to change, and always keep an open mind. EMS is a growing profession and things continue to change. Stay in tune through education, and find a mentor to help guide you. If you really want a career in EMS, go after it. This is an exciting time to be part of a changing environment.

SPECIFIC CAREER CHOICES IN EMS AS A PARAMEDIC

The field is shifting away from volunteer services toward paid professionals as the population grows and becomes more urbanized; job growth through 2012 is projected to be faster than normal. As the baby boomers age, they will require more medical services, spurring more demand for EMTs and paramedics. Additional job openings will come through attrition and stressful conditions. Volunteer and part-time jobs will be available among more rural populations. A list of common EMS job sites is listed at the end of this chapter.

FLIGHT PARAMEDIC

Working as a flight paramedic can be very rewarding. Even though you might have the chance to work as a flight paramedic right out of school, it usually takes hard work, experience, and education to land a job as a flight paramedic. Some facts about a career as a flight paramedic: There are approximately 1200 flight paramedics in the United States. To illustrate how competitive the field is, for every opening for flight paramedic, there are approximately 250 applicants. There are approximately 227 air ambulance programs in the United States. Most programs are hospital based, flying out of urban areas, and staff their helicopters with a nurse and a flight paramedic, although some use a physician and a nurse, reserving their paramedic for ground transport duties when the helicopter is grounded for weather, preventive maintenance, or other reasons.

Typical Duties of Flight Paramedics

One of the most important duties of a flight paramedic is to keep up with education. Usually, the person chosen for a flight paramedic position will already be highly trained. Most air ambulance services look for someone who came from a busy ambulance service. On top of that, they look for people who have a high degree of training. National Registry Paramedic is usually a required certification. Flight programs give great weight to those that hold instructor certifications in Advanced Cardiac Life Support (ACLS), Basic Trauma Life Support (BTLS), Pre-Hospital Trauma Life Support (PHTLS), and Pediatric Trauma Life Support (PTLS). Once on the job as a flight paramedic, your organization may require you, besides your usual requirements for continuing education, to further your education.

Another requirement of the job, not only during the interview process, but after being hired as well, is the upkeep of a professional appearance. Remember, you will be the face of the organization that you represent. You will be interacting with patients, families, other emergency professionals, doctors, and nurses. You will also be expected to assist with patient care. This can be as simple as obtaining vital signs to administering medications. This is why organizations that hire flight paramedics place such an emphasis on education, both before employment and after employment. Not only are well-educated paramedics more likely to be hired as flight paramedics, but after being hired, they are less likely to make a mistake that could jeopardize a patient. You will be expected to be an important part of the patient care team.

Typical Requirements for a Flight Paramedic

According to the International Association of Flight Paramedics, the typical requirements for a flight paramedic are as follows:

- National Registry as a paramedic
- Instructor certification in ACLS, BTLS, PHTLS, Pediatric Advanced Life Support (PALS)

- Experience in a high-volume 911 system
- Experience in interfacility transport of critical care patients
- Emergency department or hospital intensive care unit experience
- Being well-read and up-to-date on current research and treatments

To find out more information, go to the International Association of Flight Paramedics website at http://flightparamedic.org/ or http://bcctpc.org/.

CRITICAL CARE PARAMEDIC

The critical care paramedic (CCP) is expected to perform thorough assessments that include the interpretation of patient laboratory and radiological data. This advanced care usually involves transporting critically ill or injured patients from one hospital to another. CCPs' high level of decision-making and differential skills relating to patient care results in their implementing treatment measures both autonomously and after consultation with physicians.

Typical Duties of the Critical Care Paramedic

Typical duties identified in the CCP competency profile include the use of invasive hemodynamic monitoring devices and advanced techniques to manage life-threatening problems affecting patient airway, breathing, and circulation. Included is the use of ventilatory support equipment, intra-aortic balloon pumps, left ventricular assist devices, and in neonatal care, Isolette's. CCPs typically implement treatment measures that are invasive or pharmacological in nature.

TACTICAL PARAMEDIC

Specially trained tactical medicine teams often support high-risk law-enforcement operations by providing scene commanders with medical threat assessments, delivering immediate emergency medical care, and promoting the safety and health of law-enforcement personnel. Tactically trained EMS personnel achieve their objectives through mission preplanning, implementation of medically effective practices developed for law-enforcement scenarios, and provision of a critical interface between law enforcement personnel, EMS, and the emergency health-care system.

▨ Typical Duties of the Tactical Paramedic

The goals of tactical medicine are, broadly, to facilitate the success and the safety of law-enforcement missions during all phases of a tactical or SWAT operation through the delivery of preventive, urgent, and emergency medical care. The principles that are held by tactical medicine providers were initially developed by the military for small unit operations and continued to gain widespread acceptance in the civilian law-enforcement community. Their primary function during a mission is to provide broad medical oversight to operations including injury prevention, resource allocation, and rapid access to emergency medical care within the operation. During law-enforcement operations, medical activities and casualty movements are a coordinated effort between the command post, operational team leaders, and the medical support element.

A fundamental principle in tactical medicine is that the medical mission may be subordinate to the overall law-enforcement mission. In contrast to conventional EMS and hospital practices, in which the sole priority is usually the health and welfare of the patient, the essential priority in a tactical mission is the success of the law-enforcement objective. When a casualty occurs during a tactical operation, medical providers may be directed to delay or modify medical care until the tactical commander determines that rendering care will not jeopardize the overall mission.

The three goals of tactical combat casualty care are as follows:

1. Treat casualties

2. Prevent additional casualties

3. Complete the mission

The role of the tactical medic is to support the law-enforcement mission. Usually when a SWAT team takes a hit from the bad guys, more than one team member is wounded. Tactical medics care for the downed team members, the police, citizen victim, and the bad guys, too. In applying combat medicine triaging—the sorting of victims according to a system of priorities—the police are treated first because they are not a threat. Officers also have a higher survival rate because they wear body armor.

In addition to training with SWAT and going out on call-outs as members of the tactical team, tactical medics may go through weeks of basic SWAT school, a time filled with bumps, bruises, painful muscles and joints, and wagonloads of challenging stress.

Police Tactical School is not blood-in-the-mud medic training. ("Blood in the mud" refers to military combat medicine, the basis for fire and rescue tactical medicine.) Rather, tactical school is about police tactics, athletics, conquering phobias, defense and control tactics, and learning the ways of the tactical hunters, and it may include the mechanics of superior marksmanship using shotguns, handguns, automatic weapons, and less lethal launchers. Some of the tactical skills taught date back to the ancient Roman legions, whereas others are new-era tactics that use technology and unconventional ground-combat strategies.

Paramedics are transformed by the tactical school experience. Although these specialty team medics normally aren't armed with weapons, they must be proficient in their use to save their own lives or those of others. U.S. Army and Navy medics are taught to use various firearms because enemies have engaged medics and the wounded in calculated patterns of combat, targeting them with extreme acts that ignore the generally accepted codes of conventional warfare. Civilian tactical medic skills mirror those of the military. Teams do not go into situations planning that their medics will be potential shooters, but in real combat, the patterns of evolving situations are subject to change. SWAT teams are law enforcement's bedrock infantry and special operations' response to many bad situations. SWAT teams can and do save lives, prevent further violence, and bring the majority of such incidents to a peaceful conclusion.

A tactical rescue technician course prepares medics for typical scenarios. Simply transferring civilian medical care methods to the "battlefield" won't work. Tactical situations call for different medical protocols than those expected by a conventional paramedic. For example, controlling direct pressure and IV fluid applications may not be as relevant while under fire. Popular thinking also maintains that if a tourniquet is used, the patient will lose the limb. However, in reality, the most common cause of preventable combat or battlefield death has been the failure to use a tourniquet to control severe extremity bleeding. The loss of 2.5 liters of blood is likely to be associated with death from hemorrhagic shock. Indicators of shock during tactical care are the patient's state of consciousness and quality of radial pulse. Also, in combat casualty situations with open wounds, the sooner antibiotics are on board, the better. If you think you have what it takes, become a tactical paramedic.

OFFSHORE PARAMEDIC

An offshore paramedic provides emergency medical services on an offshore rig. The primary duty of an offshore paramedic is to provide first aid services to rig workers who sustain injuries, are involved in an accident, or become sick. Thus, a person must have adequate medical qualifications to become an offshore paramedic.

■ Typical Requirements

An offshore paramedic is required to hold numerous medical qualifications. The minimum requirement is usually a degree in paramedical science. This is a certificate normally issued by a state or national governing body or licensing board. Training as a military paramedic also may be acceptable. Generally, the maritime authority responsible for hiring makes the determination on a case-by-case basis regarding whether you have sufficient experience.

The "rig" medic is an essential part of an offshore rig and provides emergency medical care for all personnel, along with other various occupational health tasks. They are responsible for the provision of the rig's primary first aid response. The rig medic reports directly to the Offshore Installation Manager (OIM)/captain and chief officer.

The rig medic provides the following services and has the following responsibilities:

- Provide trauma and medical care to injured and sick personnel on the rig
- Operate and maintain the rig hospital, medical supplies, and medical equipment
- Ensure that all hospital and emergency medical equipment is serviceable and rectify any deficiencies
- Ensure the hospital and related areas are clean
- Communicate with local and/or international shore-based medical facilities as required
- Communicate with OIM/captain and safety officer with respect to injury and sickness reporting
- Advise departmental supervisors of injuries or sicknesses that involve their respective departments
- Advise OIM/master when a medical emergency evacuation of injured or sick crew member is required

DIVE PARAMEDIC TECHNICIAN

Commercial, professional, and scientific divers often find themselves at work in medical and geographic isolation. Medical evacuation of injured divers can be complicated by long distances and large bodies of water. This process may be further complicated by access difficulties, such as no runway and limited helicopter landing capabilities. Further, decompression accidents require immediate recompression. Delays in definitive treatment can result in fatal outcome, permanent neurological injury, or other career-ending complications.

Therefore, it is common to find hyperbaric recompression chambers located at the working diver's site of operation. Chambers can be aboard offshore drilling rigs, on oil and gas production platform support vessels, on research vessels, and at shore-based island marine science facilities. Treatment guidance will be directed medically by a contracted physician trained in diving medicine. However, it is uncommon for this physician to be in close proximity to the chamber and ready to evaluate the diver and accompany him or her during treatment. Rather, the contracted physician may be many hundred to several thousand miles away. To be therapeutically effective, therefore, an on-scene specialized medical presence is essential. A certified Dive Medic Technician (DMT), essentially a "diving" paramedic, represents the best option. Specialized training is necessary in order for these medics to function effectively as the eyes, hands, and ears of the diving medicine physician. Training is extended to invasive skills in order to administer physician-ordered adjunctive interventions and manage complications related to decompression insults and barotrauma.

USEFUL WEBSITES FOR FINDING AVAILABLE CAREERS IN EMS

https://www.nremt.org/

www.jems.com

http://www.emsworld.com/

http://www.firerescue1.com/

http://emsjobs.com/

www.ems1.com

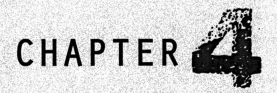

CHAPTER 4

GETTING THE JOB YOU WANT

"You will be the face of the
organization that you represent."

—*Anonymous*

WHAT IS CAREER PLANNING?

Career planning is a lifelong process, which includes choosing the right occupation (paramedicine), getting a job, growing in that particular profession, possibly changing careers, and eventually retiring. This chapter focuses on career paths in EMS as a paramedic and the process one goes through in selecting an area of expertise. This may happen once in a lifetime, but it is more likely to happen several times as we first define and then redefine ourselves and our goals.

The EMS career planning process includes four steps:

1. Self-assessment—Gather information about yourself
2. Options—Explore what area of EMS you are interested in, for example, air medicine, critical care transport, emergency 911, etc.
3. Match—During this phase of the process, you will
   a. Identify possible areas of interest
   b. Evaluate these areas (research online or trade magazines)
   c. Explore alternatives
   d. Choose both a short-term and a long-term goal

4. Action—You will develop the steps you need to take in order to reach your goal, for example,

   a. Investigating sources of additional training and education, if needed

   b. Developing a job search strategy

   c. Writing your resume

   d. Gathering company information

   e. Composing cover letters

   f. Preparing for job interviews

RESUME WRITING

Don't worry, you're not alone. Writing a resume is intimidating for everyone. What makes it difficult is knowing what to include or what not to include, what to highlight, and what to deemphasize. Human resource (HR) professionals and hiring managers may receive hundreds of resumes for any given position, and on average, they will spend about 10 to 30 seconds on yours. Organizing information incorrectly could cost you a shot at an interview and is a very common mistake made by job seekers.

Taking It to the Streets

Back when I was working as a manager for a large healthcare system in New York City, just a few months after September 11, 2001, my boss called me into his office and said, "What do you think of this?" He reaches over his desk and hands me a piece of cardboard that had a red flashing light on it. I look at him, flabbergasted, and asked, "What the @#$% is this?" He replied, "A resume!" Sure enough, I took a closer look at the hard cardboard stock, and after my heart came out of my throat, I realized, yes, a resume! This person glued his resume to cardboard stock and rigged a red flashing light with a battery to it. I guess he did this to catch the eye of the person doing the hiring. Ingenious maybe, but given the situation, it was quite scary. Needless to say, that person was not hired, and I believe the police were notified.

Making an eye-catching resume is within reason and very important, but common sense also is important. The good news is, with a little extra effort, you can create a resume that makes you stand out as a superior candidate for a job you are seeking. So, even if you face fierce competition, with a well-written resume, you should be invited to interview more often than people who might be more qualified than you.

The bad news is that your present resume is probably much more inadequate than you now realize. You will have to learn how to think and write in a style that will be completely new to you. To understand what I mean, let's take a look at the purpose of your resume. Why do you have a resume in the first place? What is it supposed to do for you? Here's an imaginary scenario. You apply for a job that seems absolutely perfect for you. You send your resume with a cover letter to the prospective employer. Plenty of other people think the job sounds great, too, and apply for the job. A few days later, the employer is staring at a pile of several hundred resumes. Several hundred, you say? Isn't that an inflated number? Not really. A job offer often attracts hundreds of resumes these days, so you will be facing a great deal of competition. Back to the prospective employer staring at the huge stack of resumes: This person isn't any more excited about going through a pile of dry, boring documents than you would be. But he has to do it, so he digs in. After a few minutes, he gets sleepy and isn't really focusing. Then, he comes across your resume. As soon as he starts reading it, he perks up. The more he reads, the more interested, awake, and excited he becomes. Most resumes in the pile have only gotten a quick glance. But yours gets read, from beginning to end. Then, it gets put on top of the tiny pile of resumes that make the first cut. These are the people who will be asked in to interview.

In this mini guide on how to write a resume, the goal is to give you the basic tools to take this out of the realm of fantasy and into your everyday life. The resume is a document with one specific purpose: to win an interview. If it does what the fantasy resume did, it works. If it doesn't, it isn't an effective resume. A resume is an advertisement, nothing more, nothing less. Research shows that only one interview is granted for every 200 resumes received by the average employer. Research also tells us that your resume will be quickly scanned, rather than read. Ten to 20 seconds is all the time you have to persuade a prospective employer to read further. Simply put, the decision to interview a candidate is usually based on an overall first impression of the resume. A quick screening that impresses the reader and convinces him of the candidate's qualifications results in an interview. As a result, the top half of the first page of your resume will either make or break you. The first few lines determine whether you have caught their interest or your resume has failed. That is why we say that your resume is an advertisement. You hope it will have the same result as a well-written ad: catch your audience's attention in a very short period of time. Imagine that you are the person doing the hiring. This person is not some anonymous paper pusher deep in the bowels of the personnel department. Usually, the person who makes the hiring decision is also the person who is responsible for operations and productivity of the agency you hope to join. This is a person who cares deeply about how well the job will be done. You need to write your resume to appeal directly to this person.

Ask yourself: What would make someone the perfect candidate for an EMS job? What does the employer really want? What special abilities would this candidate have? What would set a truly exceptional candidate apart from a merely good one? If you are not sure, you can gather hints from the job listing you are answering or ask people who work in the same company or the same EMS field. You could even call the prospective employer and ask about what the company is looking for in an employee. Don't make wild guesses unless you have to. It is very important to do this step well. If you are not addressing his real needs, he will not respond to your resume. Putting yourself in the boots of the person doing the hiring is the first, and most important, step in writing a resume that markets you, rather than describes your history or story. Every step in producing a finished document should be part of your overall intention to convey to the prospective employer that you are a truly exceptional paramedic candidate. Focus your writing efforts. Get clear and concise information about what the employer is looking for and what you have to offer before you begin your resume. Write your answers to the question "What would make someone the perfect candidate?" on notebook paper, with one answer per page. Prioritize the sheets of paper, based on which qualities or abilities you think would be most important to the person doing the hiring. Then, starting with the top priority page, fill in the rest of that page, or as much of it as you can, with brainstorming about why you are the person who best fulfills the employer's needs. Write down everything you have ever done that demonstrates that you fit perfectly with what is wanted and needed by the prospective employer.

The whole idea is to loosen up your thinking enough so that you will be able to see some new connections between what you have done and what the employer is looking for. You need not confine yourself to work-related accomplishments. Use your entire life as the palette to paint with. If Sunday School or your volunteer fire department is the only places you have had a chance to demonstrate your special gift for teaching and leadership, that's fine. The point is to cover all possible ways of thinking about and communicating what you do well. What talents do you bring to the EMS

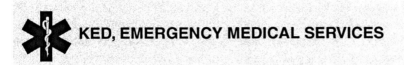

KED, EMERGENCY MEDICAL SERVICES

JOB DESCRIPTION
Work for a Leading EMS Agency

If you have passion for helping people and drive for excellence then KED-EMS is looking for you. We are looking for certified and talented Paramedics to join our team!

KED, Emergency Medical Services Agency, better known as KED, is responsible for providing excellent, pre-hospital emergency healthcare to nearly 20,000 residents in the New York metropolitan area. KED is internationally renowned for its Emergency Medical Education and Simulation Center as well as for contributing some of the leading patient outcome statistics in the nation.

Additional Details

Comprehensive Benefit Package

- $2000 Sign on Bonus
- Up to $2500 Relocation Bonus
- 10-, 12-, and 14-hour Shifts
- Health, Dental, and Vision Insurance
- State Government Retirement—Employer Matched
- 401K and 457—5% Employer Match
- Tuition Reimbursement
- $500 Employee Referral Bonus

Opportunity to Grow

- Field Advancement Opportunities
- Injury prevention team
- Special response teams (HAZMAT, Heavy Rescue, Disaster Response)

FIGURE 4-1. Sample job announcement.

market place? What do you have to offer the prospective employer? If you are making a career change or are a young person and new to the job market, you are going to have to be especially creative in getting across what makes you stand out. These brainstorming pages will be the raw material from which you craft your resume. One important part of the planning process is to decide which resume format best fits your needs. Don't automatically assume that a traditional format will work best for you. (I will provide more information about that later.)

ELEMENTS OF A RESUME

A great resume has two sections. The first section should make assertions about your abilities, qualities, and achievements. Write a powerful, but honest, advertisement that makes the reader immediately perk up and realize that you are someone special. A little advice, from a manager to a new prospective employee: Never put anything on a resume that is not true or cannot be verified.

The second section, or evidence section, is where you back up your assertions with evidence that you actually did what you said you did. This is where you list and describe the jobs you have held, your education, etc. This is all the stuff you are obliged to include.

Most resumes have only the evidence section, with no assertions. If you have trouble getting to sleep, just read a few resumes each night before going to bed. Nothing puts people to sleep better than the average resume.

The juice is in the assertions section. When a prospective employer finishes reading your resume, you want them to immediately reach for the phone to invite you in to interview. The resumes you have written in the past have probably been a gallant effort to inform the reader. You don't want them informed. You want them interested and excited.

In fact, it is best to only hint at some things. Leave the reader wanting more. Leave him with a bit of mystery. That way, he has even more reason to reach for the phone. The assertions section usually has two or three subsections. In all of them, your job is to communicate, assert, and declare that you are the best possible candidate for the job and that you are hotter than a 10-alarm fire at a gasoline refinery.

You start by naming your intended job. This may be in a separate section, titled "Objective," or may be folded into the second section, titled "Summary." If you are making a change to a new field or are a young person not fully established in a career, start with a separate objective section.

▨ The Objective

Ideally, your resume should be pointed toward conveying why you are the perfect candidate for one specific job or job title. Good advertising is directed toward a very specific target audience. When a car company is trying to sell its inexpensive compact car to an older audience, it shows grandpa and grandma stuffing the car with happy, shiny grandchildren and talks about how safe and economical the car is. When that company advertises the exact same car to the youth market, it shows the car going around corners on two wheels, with plenty of drums and power chords thundering in the background. You want to focus your resume just as specifically.

Targeting your resume requires that you be absolutely clear about your career direction or at least that you appear to be clear. If you aren't clear on where you are going, you wind up wherever the winds of chance blow you. You would be wise to use this time of change to design your future career so you have a clear target that will meet your goals and be personally fulfilling. Even if you are a little vague about what you are looking for, you cannot let your uncertainty show. With a nonexistent, vague, or overly broad objective, the first statement you make to a prospective employer says you are not sure this is the job for you.

The way to demonstrate your clarity of direction, or apparent clarity, is to have the first major topic of your resume be your objective. People who hire prospective employees remember all the jobs they applied for that they didn't really want. They know that many of the resumes they received are from people who are just using a shotgun approach, casting their seed to the winds. Then they come across a resume in the pile that starts with the following:

Objective

Dedicated professional paramedic with 17 years of patient care and teaching experience seeking a paramedic position within an organization that prides itself on exceptional patient care.

This wakes them up. They are immediately interested. This first sentence conveys some very important and powerful messages: "I want the job you are offering. I am a superior candidate because I recognize the qualities that are most important to you, and I have them. I want to make a contribution to your company." This works well because the employer is smart enough to know that someone who wants to do exactly what he is offering will be much more likely to succeed than someone who doesn't. And that person will probably be a lot more pleasant to work with as well.

Additionally, this candidate has done a good job of establishing why he is the perfect candidate in the first sentence. He has thought about what qualities would make a candidate stand out. He has started communicating that he is that person, immediately. What's more, he is communicating from the point of view of making a contribution to the employer.

Applicants are not writing from a self-centered point of view. Even when people are savvy enough to have an objective, they often make the mistake of saying something like "a position where I can hone my skill as a scissor sharpener," or something similar. The employer is interested in hiring you for what you can do for it, not for fulfilling your private goals and agenda.

Here's how to write your objective. First, decide on a specific job title for your objective. Go back to your list of answers to the question "How can I demonstrate that I am the perfect candidate?" What are the two or three qualities, abilities, or achievements that would make a candidate stand out as truly exceptional for that specific job?

The person in the above example recognized that the prospective employer prides itself in providing exceptional patient care and would be very interested in candidates that would continue and make a good representation of that organization. So the candidate made that the very first point in his resume.

Be sure the objective is to the point. Do not use fluffy phrases that are obvious or do not mean anything, such as "allowing the ability to enhance potential and utilize experience in new challenges." An objective may be broad and still somewhat undefined in some cases, such as "a mid-level management position in the EMS."

Remember, your resume will only get a few seconds of attention, at best. You have to generate interest immediately, in the first sentence the reader lays eyes on. Having an objective statement that really sizzles is highly effective. And it's simple to do.

If you are applying for several different positions, you should adapt your resume to each one. There is nothing wrong with having several different resumes, each with a different objective, and each specifically crafted for a different type of position. You may even want to change some parts of your resume for each job application. Have an objective that is perfectly matched with the job opening. Remember, you are writing advertising copy, not your life story.

It is sometimes appropriate to include your objective in the summary section rather than have a separate section for your objective. The point of using an objective is to create a specific psychological response in the mind of the reader. If you are making a career change or have a limited work history, you want the employer to immediately focus on where you are going, rather than where you have been. If you are looking for another job in your present field, it is more important to stress your qualities, achievements, and abilities first.

The Summary

The summary or summary of qualifications consists of several concise statements that focus the reader's attention on the most important qualities, achievements, and abilities you have to offer. Those qualities should be the most compelling demonstrations of why you should be hired instead of the other candidates. It gives you a brief opportunity to telegraph a few of your most sterling qualities. It is your one and only chance to attract and hold the reader's attention, to get across what is most important, and to entice the employer to keep reading.

This is the spiciest part of the resume. This may be the only section fully read by the employer, so it should be very strong and convincing. The summary is the one place to include professional characteristics that may be helpful in winning the interview. Gear every word in the summary to your targeted goal.

How do you write a summary? Go back to your lists that answer the question about what makes someone the ideal candidate. Look for the qualities the employer will care about most. Then look at what you wrote about why you are the perfect person to fill the employer's need. Choose the details that best demonstrate why the employer should hire you. Assemble it into your summary section.

The most common ingredients of a well-written summary are as follows (of course, you would not use all of these ingredients in one summary; use the ones that highlight you best):

- A short phrase describing your profession
- Followed by a statement of broad or specialized expertise
- Followed by two or three additional statements related to any of the following:
  - List of certifications
  - Unique mix of skills or specialty training
  - Range of environments in which you have experience
  - A special or well-documented accomplishment
  - A history of awards, promotions, or superior performance commendations

- One or more professional or appropriate personal characteristics
- A sentence describing professional objective or interest

Notice that the examples below show how to include your objective in the summary. If you are making a career change, your summary should show how what you have done in the past prepares you to do what you seek to do in the future. If you are a young person new to the job market, your summary will be based more on ability than experience.

■ A Few Examples of Summary Sections

- Highly motivated, professional, and career-oriented paramedic with 7 years of experience in the EMS, especially skilled at building effective, productive working relationships with patients and staff. Excellent management, negotiation, and public relations skills. Seeking a challenging position in the EMS field that offers extensive contact with the public.
- Over 10 years as an EMT with a proven track record of producing extraordinary public relations. A commitment to human compassion and community service. Energetic self-starter with excellent analytical, organizational, and creative skills.
- Healthcare professional experienced in management, program development, and policy-making in the United States, as well as in several developing countries. Expertise in EMS. A talent for analyzing problems, developing and simplifying procedures, and finding innovative solutions. Proven ability to motivate and work effectively with persons from other cultures and all walks of life. Skilled in working within a foreign environment with limited resources.
- Chief of Department, ABC Fire Company. Expertise in all areas of management, with a proven record of unprecedented accomplishment. History of the highest departmental awards. Proven senior-level experience in executive decision-making, policy direction, strategic business planning, financial and personnel management, research and development. Extensive knowledge of local government requirements in systems and equipment. Committed to the highest levels of professional and personal excellence.

■ Skills and Accomplishments

In this final part of the assertions section of your resume, you go into more detail. You are still writing to sell yourself to the reader, not to inform. Basically, you do exactly what you did in the previous section, except that you go into more detail. In the summary, you focused on your most special highlights. Now you tell the rest of the best of your story. Let the reader know what results you produced, what happened as a result of your efforts, and what you are especially gifted or experienced at doing. Flesh out the most important highlights in your summary. You are still writing to do what every good advertisement does, communicating the following: If you buy this product, you will get these direct benefits. If it doesn't contribute to furthering this communication, don't bother to say it. Remember, not too much detail. Preserve a bit of mystery. Don't tell them everything.

Sometimes the "Skills and Accomplishments" section is a separate section. In a chronological resume, it becomes the first few phrases of the descriptions of the various jobs you have held. We will cover that in a few minutes, when we discuss the different types of resumes. When it is a separate section, it can have several possible titles, depending on your situation:

- Skills and Accomplishments
- Accomplishments
- Summary of Accomplishments
- Selected Accomplishments
- Recent Accomplishments
- Areas of Accomplishment and Experience
- Areas of Expertise
- Career Highlights
- Professional Highlights
- Additional Skills and Accomplishments

There are a number of different ways to structure the "Skills and Accomplishments" section. In all of these styles, put your skills and accomplishments in order of importance for the desired career goal. If you have many skills, the last skill paragraph might be called "Additional Skills." Don't get caught in the trap that many EMS personnel do when writing a resume. Skills that are learned in paramedic school do not have to be listed under this section. Awards, citations, and highlights in your career are better than saying you are skilled in intubation, IV starting, etc.

Why Should I Hire You?

This is the first and sometimes only question I might ask you when I interview you for a job as a paramedic. How you answer this question tells me a lot about you and how you might fit into my organization. Sounds strange? Not really.

Interviewing prospective candidates for employment is a standard part of every EMS manager's job. Although there are many different types of agencies with many different types of hiring processes, the face-to-face interview is almost always part of the process at some point. In some organizations, only one person—maybe an HR specialist, maybe an EMS manager—will interview the prospective candidate; in other organizations, the interview process is a daylong affair, with the candidate meeting with several different people and groups and often participating in other evaluation methods. At my organization, each prospective paramedic takes a written knowledge examination and then meets with our medical directors, supervisors and managers, a group of peers (generally our senior paramedics), and then with me, the Administrative Director. Some candidates have described this process as excruciating, difficult, and overwhelming. Admittedly, any interview process can be these things and more, so I recommend the following strategies to help you succeed in your EMS job interview. Of course, everything you've ever read about preparing for a job interview applies here—be on time, be well rested, dress appropriately, have a well-written and up-to-date resume, etc. But, as you already know, EMS is a unique industry that, in general, demands a slightly different approach to problem solving and critical thinking than other professions.

Be Prepared for the Interview to be Challenging

Whether you're interviewing all day long or for just one hour with just one person, you need to be able to think quickly and respond to questions appropriately. This is easier said than done, for even a candidate with tremendous knowledge might be so anxious about the interview process that he or she has trouble finding the "right answers." This is especially true of those interviews where the evaluator is asking you about drug calculations, 12-lead ECG injury patterns, and other such information. It's probably a good idea to do some research about the organization you want to join and prepare for your interview by studying some issues that are meaningful to the organization. For example, my hospital's EMS service has been instrumental in improving heart attack survival in our area, and we have collaborated intensively with our emergency departments and interventional cardiology folks to help the hospital rise to be number 1 in our state for heart attack survival rate, according to national standards. I can assure you that when you sit in front of our medical directors and supervisors and paramedics, they are going to want to see how good you are with your 12-lead interpretations and approach to cardiac emergencies. Of course, this is only one example, but you should realize that any job interview is, on the part of the people in front of whom you are sitting, an expression of the organizational desire to find the person who will be most likely to fit in and meet expectations.

Be Realistic About Where You Want to Work

The EMS workplace suffers as described by the adage: "To get a good job you need experience, but to get experience you need a good job." Some organizations seek new paramedic graduates to hire. Other organizations require a minimum amount of experience before they even entertain your application. But as a new graduate, it's important to remain realistic about your expectations. Indeed, some get lucky and get the jobs they want right away. Others know in advance where they want to work and spend years biding their time to get there. Often, hospital-based services and critical care environments such as air medical programs are the most difficult organizations to get into. Municipal fire or third-service EMS agencies run the gamut from easy to difficult to enter, depending on their respective government finance and staffing needs. In many places, commercial and private ambulance services, as well as volunteer agencies, are the easiest places to get experience yet are the types of organizations most maligned by new paramedics who want badly to jump into action in an exciting environment. I have to admit that when I began working as an EMT, the first job I got was with a commercial ambulance service that primarily did interfacility transports and discharges, not as exciting as the rough and tumble world of 911 response. I had no idea where I was going to end up one day, but I did take every opportunity to learn from other EMTs and paramedics, hospital staff, physicians, or anybody else I could talk to while wrapping up those elderly patients who were being discharged to a nursing home. I am fairly certain that had I not worked for that commercial service doing those transports, I would never have been able to succeed in my career. Fundamentally, any job you get starting out is an opportunity to learn and grow, and that should be part of your plan. If that first job has to be less exciting than you expected, learning from the experience will allow you to succeed as you move ahead in your career.

Be Yourself

Very simply, a good attitude can go a very long way. I firmly believe that if you present to me as confident, willing to learn, and eager to grow in your new role, I will be more inclined to choose you over that "other guy" with 23 years of experience—and probably 23 years of bad habits! When I ask you, "Why should I hire you?" I'm looking for an idea of the kind of person and employee you might turn out to be. My medical directors and supervisors have already asked you all the difficult questions about endocrine emergencies and medication dosages. I want to know how you *feel* about working at my organization, how you *think* as an EMS professional and as a member of the EMS community, and how much you *want* to a part of that community. Of course, your first 6 or 12 months of working for me will be very telling, so here's the time to be yourself. Don't ever give a prospective employer a facade that isn't real or try to be somebody that you're not. The reality is that not every person is right for every organization, whether it be by reason of experience, organizational culture, or other environmental factors. It's as important for the new paramedic to feel comfortable and supported in his or her new role as it is for the employer to feel comfortable that the new paramedic is the right fit for the organization's needs. Both parties will be much better off if their compatibility "clicks" during the interview and can be maintained throughout the paramedic's employment. Of course, as you continue to look for growth in your career, one way you can be sure to get a good recommendation from an employer is to be yourself, be sincere, and be real.

So "Why should I hire you?" Hopefully, because you've given me every good reason: you know your paramedicine, you're enthusiastic about learning, you want to advance your career, and you are an honest, friendly person with a passion for being a paramedic. Hopefully, you can convey all of this to me at our interview, and hopefully I can be convinced that you will be a valuable member of my team. Good luck!

Daniel Meisels, MPA, EMTP, Director of EMS, UMass Memorial Medical Center, Worcester, MA

WRITING A RESUME FOR NEW EMS PERSONNEL

A resume for someone entering in the field for the first time or with less experience creates a different challenge. With a little finesse, you can still tailor your resume to be just as successful as an experienced candidate.

Objective

A one-line description of what position you're going for and with what agency. Some people say you don't need an objective. I disagree. By listing the exact job title (taken from the job description) and the agency you're testing for, I think it shows a little effort and personalization. Listing no objective is almost as bad as listing something like "to become a firefighter (and nothing else)." That makes it seem as if you use the same resume for every department. A little effort can go a long way. Also, stay away from objectives that are three to four lines long that sound like a story with no obvious ending. I've seen resumes that say something to the tune of "to obtain a position that will allow me to utilize my knowledge, skills, and abilities to be able to serve the community, and so on, and so on, and so on…." Get to the point! "To become a Firefighter for the Suffolk County Fire Department" gets your point across perfectly.

Experience

Some people like to write employment history or job history or work experience. I like experience because it is short and sweet, and because it can be paid or volunteer experience. List two to three employers at the most (don't stress—the rest are going on the application since most applications require you to list every employer you have ever worked for). Start with your present employer and work backwards (chronological order), not leaving any obvious gaps. If you are inexperienced in EMS, that's okay. List your previous employers; during an interview, the interviewer may ask you why the change in careers. Be ready to answer those types of questions. It is okay to change career paths.

Education

This section should be no more than a couple of lines. List any degrees you may possess. You need to list only one or two schools (one to two lines per school). Keep it simple. List the name of the college, the city and state of the college, the degree you received or are pursuing, and your date of graduation or expected date of application. That's it. If you graduated from college more than 10 years ago, you might want to leave that date off of the resume (it will still usually be required on the application)—just to eliminate any potential bias based on age.

Some people ask me whether they should list their units received, or all five of the colleges they've been to—including the ones they went to but never completed. I say, No. Remember—all of that information is usually requested on the application (it usually says "list every school you have ever attended"), and the resume is left up to you to pick and choose what goes on it.

Last, but not least, do not list your high school information. Why? First, that information will be going on the application. Second, it can show your age (which can be negative or positive). Even though it is illegal to discriminate on the basis of age, it can potentially happen. I'm supposed to evaluate you on the answers you provide to the questions, and that alone. If I'm on the review panel and I think you are immature, don't add fuel to the fire by announcing that you have just graduated from high school. Third, it is a waste of space. Chances are you are in college now or are taking college-level classes (EMT, Firefighter 1 Academy, etc.), so it is unnecessary.

■ Volunteer Experience

You are performing volunteer work, aren't you? Many fire departments almost expect their candidates to have some experience in volunteer or community service work. When I say community service, I don't mean the type where you put on an orange vest to do the weekend roadside cleanup work after getting convicted of a crime (not that there is anything wrong with that).

I like to list volunteer work like my experience. List the name of the organization, city and state, what exact title you have, maybe some brief duties (if you have room), and most importantly, a running tally of your total amount of volunteer hours you have performed.

■ Certificates/Licenses

Don't list all 100 of the certificates you've received. Pick about five of your most important selling points (EMT, Firefighter 1 Academy, Firefighter 1, Paramedic, CPR, Class B Firefighter's Driver's License, Rescue Systems 1, etc.). Don't list your Class D (Standard Motor Vehicle license in New York) Driver's License on the resume. It is a waste of space, and it is already on the application. Only list unique licenses that are above and beyond what the average person might possess. Which one do I list first? The one that you feel is most important, then working downwards in order of importance.

When listing each certificate or license, you only need three things:

1. Exact name/title (as taken from the certificate or license).

2. Who certified you (as taken from the certificate or license).

3. When it expires or when you took it (as taken from the certificate or license). Expiration dates are extremely important with medical-related cards such as CPR or EMT. That initial date you took the EMT class four years ago makes it look as if you were expired, if you only list the initial date you completed the class.

■ Special Skills

Do you speak, read, and/or write a second language fluently? If so, list it here. I don't know of a fire department that wouldn't want someone that was fluent in a second language. Some fire departments actually require second language fluency, in addition to EMT and Firefighter 1 just to take the entry-level firefighter test (and they get plenty of candidates).

INTERVIEWING POWER

We naturally play different roles at different times in our lives. Sometimes we are unaware of these roles because they are so much a part of our everyday lives. Effective interviewing skills require a particular role, as does working as a paramedic, being a parent, friend, spouse, dating, or playing in your favorite sport. Everyone plays various roles at different times, often in the same day; we just don't give it much thought.

Playing different roles under varying circumstances does not mean we're inauthentic; it simply means we are acting appropriately to that specific situation. A job interview isn't something we do every day; therefore, we typically have not developed an effective role for interviewing. Skilled interviewers, on the other hand, have developed techniques for being effective in their role. You're not going to win a baseball game if you don't know the rules and develop an effective role as a player.

Landing the job you want means developing this effective interviewing role; otherwise, you will likely bring other roles into play—without being aware of it—that will not be appropriate for an interview.

Being successful in any new role takes some thought and preparation. The small amount of time and effort you invest can pay significant returns in income, quality of life, and satisfaction. Here are a few interview tips:

1. Thoroughly prepare for your interviews.
   a. Present related skills, talents, and accomplishments confidently.
   b. Understand the interviewing strategies used by employers, to respond appropriately to each employer's style of interviewing and perceived requirements of the position.

    c. Use two-way communication appropriate for an interview.

    d. Prepare your questions in advance.

2. Dress appropriately. As a manager I can tell you of numerous occasions where prospective employees came to an interview in their work uniform, jeans, T-shirt. This was inappropriate and definitely someone I would not want representing the agency I managed.

3. Focus on what you can contribute to the organization rather than what the employer can do for you.

4. Don't place blame on or be negative about past employers. This is a big no-no.

5. Follow up strategically after each interview.

Types of Interviews

1. Telephone Interview

Telephone interviews are becoming more common. They save the employer time and indicate whether a face-to-face interview is warranted. Telephone Interviews are typically used to make a preliminary assessment of a candidate's qualifications.

2. Panel Interview

In a panel interview, typically three to six members in different roles in the organization ask candidates questions to assess their knowledge, skills, team fit, ability to make decisions, etc.

3. Videoconference Interview

Videoconference Interviews are becoming more common. They expand the scope of searching for qualified candidates with less cost and time involvement.

4. Reverse-Role Interview

In the reverse-role interview, the interviewer is unprepared, short on time, hurried, distracted, or simply unskilled at interviewing. The result is that the interviewer does not ask the appropriate questions—without which he or she may not understand your ability to perform successfully or other factors that indicate you are a good fit.

5. Informal Interview

An informal interview is casual and relaxed; it is intended to induce candidates to talk comfortably so that they will reveal more information than they might otherwise. Your privacy is important to remember at this point: too much information too soon could screen you out from consideration.

6. Layered-Questions Interview

A layered-questions interview is common among skilled interviewers. The interviewer asks a series of questions, often overlapping, designed to gather information and find discrepancies in a candidate's answers.

7. Stress Interview

A stress interview is generally intended to put a candidate under stress to assess his or her reactions. Once a candidate demonstrates that he or she can perform effectively under stress, the test is passed.

8. Performance Interview

In a performance interview, the interviewer asks candidates to role-play job functions to assess their knowledge and skills. (This is not the same as a case interview, in which it typically is only a portion of the interview and is focused on performance or knowledge rather than critical thinking.)

9. Case Interview

The case interview is a special type of interview commonly used by management-consulting firms and is increasingly being used in many other organizations. It helps the interviewer analyze your critical-thinking skills. If you are not familiar, do not have experience, or are not comfortable with case analysis, it can be one of the most difficult interviews to endure.

In a case interview, a candidate is given a problem to see how he or she would work it out on the spot. The problems that are presented come in many forms, but the interviewer wants to assess the candidate's analytical skills, ability to think under pressure, logical thought process, business knowledge and acumen, creativity, communication, and quantitative analysis skills.

10. Assessment Instruments (Tests)

"Get used to it!" You're now in a profession that requires not only written exams, but practical exams as well. This will probably follow you throughout your career in EMS. Don't fret! The more confident, experienced, and knowledgeable you become, the more you realize a lot of exams are presented in the same format. Employers use various types of assessments (commonly referred to as *tests* or *inventories*) to determine whether you are a likely fit. Among these are the following:

- Personality inventory (assesses personality types)
- Aptitude inventory (assesses aptitudes in certain skill areas)
- Interest inventory (assesses interests in various occupational categories)
- Combination instruments (combines any of the above)

- Knowledge inventory
- Skills inventory

Salary discussions during an interview focus on what you have made in prior positions and/or what you are seeking to earn in your next position. (The rules are different if you're responding in writing to a written request for a salary history or requirements from an advertised position.)

Follow-up can significantly affect whether an offer is extended. Following up after an interview addresses a key employer concern, which is your interest level in the position. In addition, you are demonstrating, by the very act of following up, personal and professional qualities that are typically sought by an employer: dedication, tenacity, attention to detail, and the ability to follow through. In some instances, employers may even use the lack of follow-up as a screening device: a way to narrow down the number of candidates to a short list; those who do follow up become finalists.

More often, however, there are usually several top candidates, each with various tradeoffs regarding strengths and liabilities. The employer is often faced with a difficult decision; and follow-up, when handled correctly, offers a strategic means of tipping the scales in your favor. Besides demonstrating your interest level and the desired qualities employers seek, strategic follow-up offers the opportunity to reassure the employer regarding any concerns he or she might have about you being the best choice for the position. This can make the difference between an offer being extended to you rather than another candidate. Even if an offer is not extended to you at this particular time, it helps you to stand out—and could lead to another position in the future.

There are several ways to follow up and you may want to let your interest level in each position guide you. Thank-you cards and follow-up letters are most common. Thank-you cards create an opportunity to reconnect with the interviewer, remind him or her of your unique skills and accomplishments, and reiterate your interest in the open position. Strategic follow-up letters are considerably more effective; however, they require a little more effort on your part. These letters can be sent via e-mail or postal mail. Strategic follow-up strengthens the interviewer's perception of you and addresses any concerns you felt the interviewer might have about this position being the right fit for you. It also provides an opportunity to add any related skills, abilities or interests, and other information that you did not think of during the interview, which may have a bearing on your candidacy. Because typically there will be several top candidates for the position, each with various tradeoffs regarding strengths and liabilities, this follow-up helps nudge that often difficult decision in your favor.

Immediately after the interview, it is essential to write down particulars. Include the details of the job description as described by the interviewer, as well as specific information regarding the company and department in which you would be working and any skills for which you felt the interviewer had a concern. Keep in mind that although follow-up can make the difference in being extended an offer now, it also helps to leave doors open for the future; interviewing for one position may lead to another.

CHAPTER 5

TAKING THE CLASSROOM TO THE STREETS!

WHAT IS IT REALLY LIKE TO BE A PARAMEDIC?

To this day, I will never forget my first EMS run, right out of EMT class and newly certified. My volunteer fire department was toned out for an imminent birth at one of our houses that operate as a single room occupancy. While responding, I kept thinking, "I'll never be able to do this." My face blanched. I turned nauseated and hot. I thought I would pass out. Too ashamed to look up, I sat there in the passenger seat wondering if I would be able to perform the necessary skills to deliver a baby and take care of mom and the new-born baby. Worse, what happens if they really needed my help? Well, after 20+ years as an EMS provider, I realize how fortunate I was to have good instructors, good mentors, and most of all the ambition to go beyond what the EMS textbooks had to offer and continue educating myself, every day. By the way, the baby and mother did well.

So, what's it *really* like to be a paramedic? Is it glitz and glamour, and rushing in and saving lives and being revered? I would have to say "no"; unfortunately, that is fantasy world or Hollywood, which many expect and few are aware of. In fact, much of being a paramedic involves downtime, station and truck duties, communication skills, being able to cooperate with others, and enduring many sleepless nights.

What is your greatest fear as a new paramedic?

Being unsure of myself during a pediatric arrest, and having to deal with grieving family members!

—*Thomas Hoar, Paramedic (2 months)*

I can probably speak for most EMS professionals, new or seasoned. One of the most difficult calls we will respond to in EMS is a critical pediatric call. EMS calls involving pediatric patients are emotionally charged and can generate a high level of stress for the personnel who respond. Apprehension, uneasiness, and anxiety are common in calls that involve pediatric patients. The best way to control this fear and anxiety is to educate, train, and perform real-life-like scenarios. Have personnel act as the parents or family members, use mannequins that are used for intubation, IV starting, intraosseous, and become familiar with protocols and the Broselow tape.

A few months back, I responded to a 2-year-old hanging. The chief arrived on the scene and summoned the ambulance to the scene forthwith. Apparently, the child was left unattended for 5 minutes, and when the father reentered the room, he found his son hanging from the chain attached to the vertical blinds. When we arrived, the father was performing CPR frantically, crying for us to help. There were some responders who were really traumatized by this. Ultimately, we resuscitated the child and transported him to the hospital. He died 2 days later from an anoxic brain injury from the hanging. This was my 19th or 20th pediatric arrest. That's in my entire career. If you average it out, it comes out to one a year. So it is extremely important to maintain your skills and protocol knowledge, and train, train, train.

My biggest fear in finishing medic class and being a new medic is starting the career itself. There seems to be more and more medic courses being offered with many EMTs wanting a job in the emergency sector, but a small amount of positions open.

—*Louis Brand, EMT-Paramedic student*

This statement by Louis is very true. The best way to make yourself stand out among the paramedic population when it comes to landing a job is to market yourself. Advertise your ability in your resume. Interview, interview, interview! And last but not least, continue your education. More and more employers are looking for EMS personnel who not only have the paramedic license or certification but also have some form of college or formal education. As the profession progresses and matures so to speak, you will have to become marketable by having specialty training and education, skills that set you at the top of the list.

The healthcare system is such that paramedics are called in increasingly alarming numbers, from everything from a stubbed toe to constipation. How did it get so off-kilter? First, from my own observations, it seems that we have encouraged increased dependency indirectly by making the 911 system available and widely promoting it. Second, the incidence of liability for medical staff has had the deleterious effect of deferring all clients to EMS, instead of conferring with them either in person or over the phone. Third, and perhaps the most distressing, is the unwritten acknowledgment that by going to the hospital by ambulance means that the individual is much more likely to get past the waiting room at the emergency department and be seen. These people are often referred to as "frequent fliers," and they know the game well.

Thus, many of the calls paramedics respond to turn out to be nonemergencies. On average, 90% of the runs made with lights and sirens are either manufactured complaints or non-life-threatening events.

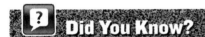

Did You Know?

According to the New York City Fire Department EMS, in 2009, NYC EMTs and paramedics responded to 1,236,730 incidents. Of those, 791,810 were classified as non-life-threatening medical emergencies.[1]

I have personally gone several shifts responding to low-priority calls before actually receiving a true emergency. I tell you this because the incidence of burnout for a paramedic is high. The monotony of running calls that are not emergencies, especially throughout the night, have a wearing effect. Many people develop dark humor and resent having to do so much unnecessarily. Driving all over town for 24 hours is tiring, as well as wearing on the body. Being a paramedic is also disrupting to your sleep patterns. Working 24-hour shifts means that one might be up the entire night, and it is true for some. If the person has a family or another job on the side, it increases stress and affects moods. It wears down the immune system and encourages bad eating and drinking habits. Being tired means a person will less likely take care of himself or herself by exercising, which only exacerbates stress. Being exposed to a variety of communicable diseases is also commonplace. Methicillin-resistant *Staphylococcus aureus* (ie, MRSA)

1   New York City Fire Department. Available at: http://www.nyc.gov/html/fdny/html/home2.shtml. Accessed December 30, 2010.

infections, viral infections, hepatitis, tuberculosis, and human immunodeficiency virus (HIV) are only some of the viruses lingering about. There is added danger in that one might accidentally get poked with the same needle used in a carrier of one of these viruses. Who can say what is crawling on a uniform that is taken home and placed in the family laundry?

Many injuries are associated with lifting, something we are subjected to almost every shift. It is no doubt that people are growing bigger and bigger. Many of them are bed-bound and cannot help themselves. Some are on the floor and weigh 300 pounds or more. Picking up a body is nothing like lifting weights in a gym. It moves, shifts, and even grabs you as you try to move it. Injuries can put a person out of work for months at a time. The compensation is nil compared to the price paid for getting oneself hurt. Oh yeah, I failed to tell you that they are usually "carry downs" from every other floor but the ground level.

Paramedics also have carbon monoxide exposure. Did you know that people who work out of vehicles have on average a 10% higher CO content in their bloodstream? We unknowingly breathe exhaust fumes. Much of being a paramedic is riding in and working around running vehicles.

Yet, having taken much of the glamour out of being a paramedic, I would like to add at this point that we do save lives. Most "saves" are done to people who are chronically ill and others who are battling terminal illness. However, there is nothing like using your training and really seeing it work. This is why people decide to become paramedics. Isn't that why you became a medic? The few times this is experienced makes up for all the other stuff we have to deal with. The pay is nominal. You are not going to get rich being a paramedic. It is unfortunate but true. The pay is the satisfaction of knowing that you are making a difference, even if it is in a small measure. The experience gained is also valuable and can lead to higher career choices later. The repeated stress of being under the gun, so to speak, is also very valuable in terms of being able to handle a variety of situations and making snap decisions. If gone into with realistic expectations, EMS can be a stimulating and satisfying field.

Self-gratification is what I like most about my career as a paramedic. Knowing I helped countless people throughout my career is what makes me stay in the field. No, it's not the CPR save where the person goes on living on a ventilator the rest of his or her life! It is the asthmatic or ST-elevation myocardial infarction patient, or maybe it is the depressed elderly woman who I made smile. That is what this job is all about. Really! If you think you can come in and make save after save, I can guarantee that you won't be here in 2 years. Being a paramedic requires patience and of course patients. I recall looking back to when I was a new paramedic in the South Bronx, thinking I was going to save the world, just to find out that not every patient requires

Advanced Life Support (ALS) intervention. A lot of what we do is understanding what is going on, deciphering a history, making a possible treatment plan, and most of all transporting the patient to the correct receiving facility. My biggest suggestion to a new paramedic would be to find someone who is a good mentor, who will guide you through the ins and outs of being a paramedic. Someone you trust and someone who trusts you. Ask questions, not only to your mentor, but also to the doctors as well. Follow up on cases that were and weren't so clear-cut, and review them with the doctors in the emergency department. Knowledge is not only power, but it is also lifesaving as well. My next suggestion is to never listen to someone who says, "This is the way we do it in the streets." That is the wrong answer in my book. Everything you learn in the classroom gives you a solid foundation. Are there ways that can be used in the street to make assessment or treatment easier? Absolutely, but do as you are trained. Shortcuts can be used when you have a handle on what is needed to be a paramedic. By the way, after many years and thousands of calls, I still use what I was taught in medic school. I guarantee that your instructor won't steer you wrong. I still do concentric circles when cleaning an IV site. Something my lab instructor drilled into our heads every day. These concepts of good patient care are forever burned in my head. Or maybe it was the drug calculation math? Desired dose/dose on hand = volume to be administered!

 ## Taking It to the Streets

It's funny how different people are when it comes to school and work. As I sit here and write this portion of the *Paramedic Survival Guide*, there is a blizzard outside. Really, I'm not making this up! I am working a 16-hour shift waiting for the "big one" to come in. And not only are we expecting 16-in of snow, they are also saying the wind gusts are 60 to 65 mph. I am sitting here with a medic student who is going to graduate in a few months; he is all sorts of mad because he has to commute in the morning to a hospital emergency department rotation, maybe 12 miles away. I look back at my medic school days, commuting from Long Island to Brooklyn, Queens, "The Bronx," and Manhattan. Each way was 60 to 65 miles. Rain, sleet, snow, it didn't matter. Alright, I know it sounds like a U.S. Postal Service commercial. The students of the class wouldn't dare "bang out" (ie, call in sick) because of bad weather. Yeah, I know it sounds like your mother or father, when they went to school barefoot, uphill, blah, blah, blah! The reality is, for every seat in our class (NYC-EMS Paramedic Program), there were four to five people willing to take our spot. Medic school was very competitive to get into. My point is that people truly rely on us to respond to their emergencies. This includes both our employer and the patient. Regardless of the situation at hand, poor weather, or our own personal problems, people rely us when they are in a time of need. Take pride in your job! Give yourself extra time to get to work. Nobody says this job is easy. On September 11, 2001, I was away from my family for 2 weeks, with no clothes, the uncertainty that something else would happen, and a list of close friends that were just murdered. I am not saying that this is an everyday occurrence, but you never know what your next call will be.

Let me ask you one question. Don't look behind you. I am talking to you. Think about this for a minute. You're driving your car, and suddenly, *BANG!* Out of nowhere, a tractor trailer crashes into you. You're pinned in your car, life flashing before your eyes. You say to yourself, this is it! The medics and fire department work feverishly to disentangle you from the wreck. You go unconscious.... A moment later, you wake up in the emergency room and hear the nurse say, "What are we going to do? This kid needs a thoracic surgeon!" From the other side of the room, you hear the unit clerk say, "He called in because the weather is bad!" Get my drift? Don't pick up bad habits from people who think they know the "system."

TOP 10 "HOT" TIPS FOR NEW PARAMEDICS

1. **Know your protocols**. Field training is a great time for learning, but it isn't a time for learning protocols. By knowing your protocols before you get into the field, you give yourself the opportunity to use your field training to learn how to apply the protocols to the various situations found in the field.

2. **Make a list**. Knowing your strengths and weaknesses both in knowledge and in clinical skills is important. Understand that weaknesses are not failures; rather, they are merely areas with room for improvement. They are areas that we are often afraid to examine but can be the sources of our greatest successes once we master them. By knowing what you need to work on, you can focus on specific learning situations with your patients, preceptor, and training officers.

3. **Communicate efficiently.** This is simple yet complex and easy to do but easy to blunder. We hear only half of what is said to us, understand only half of that, believe only half of that, and remember only half of that. So listen to what people say—patients, mentors, or coworkers. To improve your communication, recognize the importance of listening. It saves time, cuts through people's defenses, and you get more information without having to repeat the conversation. Communication also involves body language. We communicate through body language sometimes more than we do with words.

4. **Facilities.** Know what facilities in which you have to work within your region and the approximate transport time to each from your dispatch area. Be aware of any specialty centers where local hospitals can handle trauma, burns, pediatric, or maternity patients. Also, you may consult with a different facility than the one to which you transport. Be aware of which hospitals can give you online medical direction and which ones can't. Some providers transport to nearby, out-of-jurisdiction hospitals but have to consult with a different, in-state hospital.

5. **Use a mirror.** Professionalism starts with your appearance. You want to make a good first impression to your patients. Take a moment and make sure you look like the professional EMS provider you have spent so much time training to become. If you need it, take the time to get a haircut. Don't forget to brush your teeth and carry some breath mints in your pocket for those long shifts when you don't get a chance to brush. There are no second chances for first impressions.

6. **Ask questions.** A paramedic's job is to learn. That's it, pure and simple. Ask questions before a call, during a call, and after a call. Good paramedic mentors will make sure there is time for you to ask questions and debrief after calls, but they may assume you don't need this after every routine call. If you have questions, ask them. Every EMS provider has seen things that others have not, and the only way to share that information is to ask each other questions about how patients presented on a certain call or how a transport worked out.

7. **"I don't know!"** These are three simple words that make you human, and nothing else. They are not a sign of failure, but of a willingness to learn. Saying these words to your mentor or field training officer means you are putting patient care first and your ego second. If you stumble along through a call without asking for help when you need it, you will seem like a poor, ill-prepared EMS provider. Mentors and training officers will think that you were doing the wrong things on purpose or were skipping important steps in patient care out of laziness. Put what you have learned

from your education first. Learn to properly ask for help, and don't be afraid to say "I don't know" when you encounter untried territory. It's the sign of a superior provider.

8. **Review.** Along with making a list of strengths and weaknesses, asking questions, and saying "I don't know" comes reviewing at home after a difficult or problematic call. Pull out your class notes and textbooks to review recommended practices. Talk with your mentor after the call and then again the next day after you have reviewed in order to get your questions answered. Ongoing education is part of every medical field. From EMTs to physicians, all of us have to constantly go back to the classroom or read journals to refresh our knowledge and gain new education. It's part of the job and part of being a professional.

9. **Newer is not better.** New EMS providers often enter the field setting with a great deal of enthusiasm and knowledge. They can't wait to put that knowledge to use. Sometimes, they will see their instructor, preceptor, or another provider offer an alternative solution to a given situation that is the old way to do things. Be respectful of those who have gone before you. Just because it's the old way doesn't mean it's wrong. Take the time to learn several methods for getting a job done. You will soon learn that every call, every patient, and every situation is different. Knowing two ways to, for example, splint a broken bone may save your butt someday.

10. **Have Fun!** Getting into the field for the first time is the beginning of the rest of your EMS career. Enjoy your first moments on the street. Make sure you remember how you felt on that first call, after that first successful IV, medication push, or radio consult. Try to keep some of that enthusiasm in your back pocket for those times later in your career when you've had a bad day. It will remind you of why you are doing this job and you'll be thankful for it!

EMS TRICKS OF THE TRADE

Most of us were taught to start our IVs bevel-up, but when you're trying to thread a plastic catheter into a little vein, quite often the leading edge of your trocar pierces the opposite wall of the vein before you're ready to advance the catheter. There you are, with needle in the vein and catheter still outside it. Perhaps you try to shallow the angle of your needle and advance a bit, and as often as not, you see the hematoma form at the same time you notice flashback in the catheter hub. If you've ever had that happen to you, try inserting your IV catheters bevel-down. Doing so will make the angle of insertion much more shallow, thus minimizing the chance of poking the very end of that needle through the opposite wall before the tip of your cannula enters the lumen of the vein.

It's an old trick that was first taught to me by a neonatal fellow in my Critical Care Training Program at Columbia Presbyterian NICU. It takes some practice, and with certain types of protective IV catheters, more than a little gymnastics, but the technique can be mastered with all types of protective catheters. Or, if you prefer, keep a few of the old, non-protected IV catheters on hand especially for this purpose.

If tiny veins in pediatric patients—or, for that matter, geriatric patients—always make you pause, consider using the bevel-down IV technique. If you have access to an IV therapy manikin, practice the technique on it. You may find it a useful trick one day.

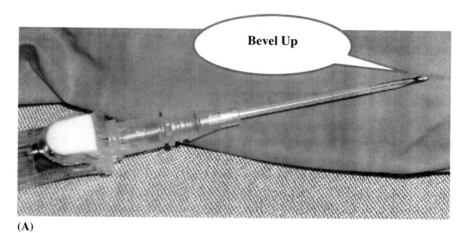

(A)

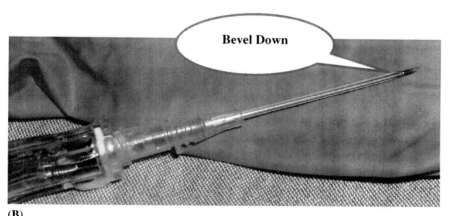

(B)

FIGURE 5-1. Intravenous catheters with bevels up (A) and down (B). *(Photos by Peter A. DiPrima Jr.)*

TREATING "STEAKHOUSE SYNDROME"

Steakhouse syndrome, otherwise known as an esophageal food bolus obstruction, is a medical emergency occurring when a foreign body becomes stuck in the esophagus. Standard treatment in-hospital includes endoscopy, digestive enzymes (such as papain), or glucagon. An interesting property of glucagon is that it has smooth muscle properties when given intravenously.

A 1.0-mg glucagon slow IVP under medical direction may be an effective means of terminating any spasms and passing the obstruction. Glucagon could also be considered in the case of a recent clearing of a foreign body airway or esophageal obstruction with excessive coughing or spasms. Unfortunately, the use of glucagon in the field to treat true esophageal food bolus obstructions is limited by an inability to conduct radiological studies, so unless transport times are long or the EMS system rural, safe and expeditious transport should not be delayed.

MANAGING THE INTUBATED PATIENT

End-tidal CO_2 waveform capnography is truly a standard of care throughout the nation and is used to confirm and continually monitor intubated patients.[2] A trick in limiting flexion and hyperextension of a patient's neck and airway is to apply a cervical collar and immobile his or her head and spine to a long backboard after intubation. This process reduces movement on the obvious trauma patient and reduces movement in the intubated medical patient. This significantly reduces the possibility of the endotracheal tube from being dislodged during transport and patient movement.

Tips and Tricks

- When a patient is placed on a backboard (long spine board), take a blood pressure cuff and place the bladder under his or her lower back. Inflate the cuff until the patient feels comfort in the lumbar region of the back.

---

2 American Heart Association. Highlights of the 2010 American Heart Association Guidelines for CPR and ECC.

- While extricating a patient down a flight of stairs using a stair chair who has an IV line in place, use a hemostat or karabiner; run it through the hole in the top of the IV bag and clip it onto your shirt lapel. This will keep the IV bag out of the way and keep the IV line flowing.

- When knocking on a door, make it a habit to stand to the side of the door. If you do it every time, you will instinctively do it on a call where it might save your life.

- Tape a soft-tip suction catheter to the laryngoscope blade. The catheter hole to control suction is taped to where your thumb is when holding the handle. During intubation, you can suction at the exact time and location needed to visualize the cords. Caution: You are going to need to work on how to tape the tube to the blade. Practice on a manikin to ensure your suction catheter and tape don't block your vision; it took me a few tries during practice before I figured it out. A key to success is to put the catheter tube to the outside of the blade. Put the tape flat so it doesn't cover your vision down the inside of the blade.

NEEDLE DECOMPRESSION

Attaching a stopcock to the end of the angiocatheter serves as a means to control the "venting" of the pneumothorax (by using a stopcock to shrink the size of the pneumothorax). Start with the pneumothorax venting to the outside air. Next, have the patient take a forceful breath out. This maximizes the intrathoracic pressure and vents the pneumothorax air out through the stopcock. Then close the stopcock. When the patient breathes in, the outside air can no longer be sucked back into the intrathoracic cavity. After several rounds of this timed inhalation-exhalation routine with the stopcock, your patient should feel significantly better.

AUSCULTATION OF LUNG SOUNDS

Prehospital providers seem to have trouble listening to lung sounds. Many instructors have told me that this is an "art form." Here are a couple of useful tricks to help reduce external noise. First, place your stethoscope in the axilla of the armpit, and then have the patient cover it with his or her arm. This will reduce almost all of the external noise.

INTUBATION

Tip 1: Grip site along laryngoscope handle. Variable force is necessary to lift the tongue and pharyngeal soft tissue anteriorly in order to visualize the vocal cords during intubation. For patients with excessive neck soft tissue, a large tongue, or trismus, the operator may need to exert significant force to obtain an unobstructed view. To minimize exertional trembling by the hand holding the laryngoscope, grasp the laryngoscope handle as close to the blade as possible. This gives you the greatest control and strength.

Tip 2: Endotracheal tube lubrication. Occasionally, the endotracheal tube may become "caught up" along a floppy epiglottis. Because it is difficult to predict when this may happen, prelubricate the tube tip with a thin layer of water-soluble lubricant, such as K-Y jelly. This lubricant can also minimize the degree of surface trauma to the trachea and tracheal rings as the tube passes through the vocal cords.

PREHOSPITAL ETHICAL ISSUES

The single most important question a paramedic has to answer when faced with an ethical challenge is: What is in the patient's best interest?

Over the past 30 years, the field of prehospital medicine has undergone impressive growth. As the body of knowledge continues to grow, as more technology is introduced, and as research defines and refines the uniqueness of prehospital emergency medical care, the challenges of the prehospital setting are becoming more than operational and medical. Efficient response, appropriate care, and safe, expeditious transport are the expectant fundamental components of prehospital care. However, more and more prehospital providers are facing challenging ethical dilemmas.

The prehospital provider must frequently interact and negotiate with reluctant patients; counsel those patients who ask for advice or refuse care; address requests for limitation of resuscitation; assume some degree of personal risk in the care of agitated, uncooperative, or infectious patients; deal with social and psychiatric challenges; and respond to a variety of unusual requests that may not be medical in nature. Each of these situations presents potential ethical conflicts. Formal training alone does not prepare the prehospital provider to deal with ethical situations. Many learn by experience, whereas some are guided by well-defined policy. Appropriate resolution of ethical dilemmas in prehospital care is promoted when those who provide and those who direct prehospital care are educated and sensitive to ethical conflicts that may arise.

Resuscitation Efforts

EMS should be available to all persons in need, including terminally ill patients who need to be transported to the hospital for palliative care. Prehospital care providers require a means to honor patient directives to limit intubation and avoid application of cardiopulmonary resuscitation (CPR). This issue often presents a complex problem. Requests to limit resuscitation will confront the provider in many forms. Written Do-Not-Resuscitate (DNR) orders, living wills, clear and unequivocal family requests, and a relative's impulsively expressed reservations about life support will be encountered. Acceptable directives must guarantee that withholding resuscitation would reflect the informed wishes of competent patients.

Reliable mechanisms have been developed by some EMS systems to identify patients in the prehospital setting who do not want to be resuscitated. These items allow recognizable, consistent, legally accepted written statements to be used as valid indication that the patient wishes to have no CPR or intubation at the time of cardiac arrest. The goal is to minimize ambiguity and maximize patient autonomy. Such documents must be familiar to the EMT or paramedic, be easily recognizable, and be specific in regard to the interventions to be withheld. Extensive written lists should be avoided, since the time to read, interpret, determine the applicability, and decide on a course of action threaten appropriate care. There can be no delay or question when such directives are presented. Some states have passed statutes to authorize prehospital orders to limit resuscitation. Verbal requests by relatives cannot be accepted. When ordinary verbal requests are made, it is not clear that they represent the informed decision of the patient. An exception to this rule exists when the relative holds a durable power of attorney to make healthcare decisions. The person who holds power of attorney for healthcare decisions has a duty to base decisions on the patient's values and wishes; the decision-maker must assess what the patient would have wanted. As a legally recognized proxy decision-maker for the patient, this person may request that resuscitation be withheld. Based on this direction, resuscitation ethically can be withheld. This might present confusion for prehospital care providers who have little experience in dealing with these situations or who may be unsure whether the decision has been well thought out. Even a legally designated proxy decision-maker may make impulsive requests that are not carefully thought through. Prehospital care providers should not enter into what may be a complicated and uncomfortable discussion regarding healthcare options and questions of the legitimacy of withholding resuscitation. At the time of crisis in the prehospital setting, such discussions are not appropriate. If there is any doubt about the legitimacy or authority of a request to withhold resuscitation, appropriate resuscitation maneuvers *must* be initiated. If the authority is clear and the EMS acknowledges such directives, there is no ethical reason that they could not be accepted. Optimal communication is facilitated through a written "no CPR/no intubation" order that is familiar and acceptable to the prehospital care provider.

"Dead on arrival" (DOA) policies specify those patients who should not undergo resuscitation attempts, because the effort would be futile. Although the medical criteria that define futility must be discussed from a scientific point of view, the ethical implications are evident. Prehospital care providers may be biased regarding age, underlying illness, or other factors that may or may not suggest futility. In general, age, medical history, social position, or patient vices should not determine whether resuscitation is initiated. The values and attitudes of the paramedic must not enter into such decisions. The decision to determine that a patient is "dead on arrival" must be made on the basis of firm scientific grounds. In those medical conditions that have been scientifically accepted as futile, resuscitation should not be performed. Strict criteria, education, and appropriate supervision and review must be part of a DOA policy. Examples include extreme dependent lividity, tissue decomposition, rigor mortis, decapitation, or similarly mortal injuries.

▓ Patient Confidentially

When should providers speak with the press? Should they speak with police regarding intoxicated patients? Should they ever be concerned about broadcasting names over radiofrequencies that can be monitored by the public? Are prehospital care providers appropriately sensitive regarding the confidentiality of a patient's medical diagnoses? Numerous threats to patient confidentiality exist in the routine of prehospital care. In a very short time, prehospital care providers become privileged to sensitive information. Indiscriminate discussion or inappropriate release of the information could present both ethical and legal threats. All information that is encountered by prehospital personnel must be considered privileged and treated as confidential. Information should be communicated only to those who are assuming direct care of the patient and who have similar obligations of confidentiality. The only information that should be discussed over the radio is that which is necessary to provide for optimal care of the patient.

Casual conversations should be avoided with parties uninvolved in the care of the patient. Discussion of cases that do not identify the patient and are used for educational purposes present no ethical conflict. Clear policy and appropriate education are important to promote the highest standards of prehospital care.

The Bad-News Bearer, the Toughest Job in EMS

Despite that death is a basic truth of our profession, we are usually woefully unprepared to explain it to those left behind. Regardless of how peaceful or traumatic the circumstance, I do not know of anyone who enjoys doing a death notification. They get the heck out of Dodge; that's the deeply rooted sense of emotional self-preservation that wants us to avoid being snarled in whatever the grief-laden aftermath is going to be.

Did You Know?

Did you know that more than 43,000 people die in the United States from motor vehicle crashes each year? That more than 35,000 people commit suicide? That more than 16,000 die from falls? That more than 17,000 die by homicide? Together, more than 150,000 North Americans die each year as a result of sudden, violent death. Oh yeah, did I mention cardiovascular disease? 1,000,000 people each year.

Death is never easy, but for families and friends affected by sudden death, grief is especially traumatic. Deaths caused by accidents, homicide, and suicide typically seem premature, unjust, and very, very wrong. Obsessive thoughts and feelings about what the death must have been like for the person who died and what might have been done to prevent it often color the grief process. Strong feelings of anger and regret are also common. Understanding and expressing these feelings helps survivors; over time and with the support of others, they come to reconcile their loss.

Although awareness of the necessity of death notification education has increased, it has yet to be translated into a readily available curriculum. That does not mean we should remain ignorant of the impact we can have upon the survivors of loss. With a little education and some insight, there are definitive steps you can take in your approach that can help at least mitigate some of the emotional devastation and shock you are otherwise taking part in delivering. Remember that the deceased is not your only patient; in fact, he or she is no longer the priority. The loved ones at the scene are also your responsibility, and your choice of words and actions will leave an irrevocable mark on their memory.

"Life is a fatal condition, with a 100% chance of mortality."

—Anonymous

Notification of Death

Notification of death presents unique difficulties for both paramedic personnel and survivors. Both notifying and being notified of the death of a loved one are most often painful and extremely traumatic experiences. Although there is no "good" way to notify survivors of a sudden and unexpected death, the compassionate expression of dignity and respect will result in proper notification that will help survivors cope with their great loss.

It is recommended that paramedics, preferably those involved in the care, notify the next of kin of the death. At no time should survivors be notified of the death by telephone. It is further suggested that agencies utilize two EMS personnel to effectuate the in-person notification function, and that they be in uniform. Although some survivors have asserted that the appearance of a uniformed individual at their home caused trauma, the uniform itself is an identification that will prevent confusion. Thus, the survivors will be more likely to be put at ease. Also, there are other advantages in utilizing two EMS personnel to extend a death notification. One medic should communicate the information while the other carefully observes the reactions of the survivors. Individuals react to death in various and often unexpected ways. Some may suffer physical reactions that may require emergency care, whereas others may become violent or aggressive, which may require their being physically restrained from harming themselves or others. In addition, it may be advantageous to notify two or more survivors separately, especially in instances that may require them to provide law enforcement officers with investigative information.

"I've learned that people will forget what you said, people will forget what you did, but people will never forget how you made them feel."

—Dr. Maya Angelou

If possible, the notifying EMS personnel should obtain pertinent medical information about the survivors prior to making the notification. This will allow the notifying paramedics to respond more properly to the immediate needs of those who suffer chronic medical problems such as heart disease, hypertension, etc.

When speaking to the patient's survivors, the medics should introduce themselves and politely request that any children be brought into a different room. The medics should attempt to seat the survivors and ensure that the notification be made to the appropriate individuals. The medics should inform the survivors of the death simply and directly and answer their questions tactfully but honestly. They should provide as much information as possible. The paramedics should ask the survivors if they would like to have family or friends contacted to assist them. Under no circumstances should the medics depart the residence of a survivor who resides alone until a designated friend or relative arrives.

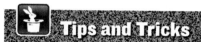

HELPFUL PHRASES

I can't imagine how difficult this is for you.

I know this is very painful for you.

I'm so sorry for your loss.

It must be hard to accept.

It's harder than most people think.

You must have been very close to him/her.

How can I help?

Most people who go through this react just as you are.

After the survivors have recovered from the initial shock of learning of the loss of a loved one, the medics should explain what can be expected of them in the immediate future. The survivors should be informed that it may be necessary for them to identify the deceased. If so, EMS should transport or arrange the transportation of the survivors to and from the hospital or morgue through the use of law enforcement. Survivors should also be informed that certain laws may require that an autopsy be performed to establish the exact cause of death. If it appears likely that survivors will have to be questioned by law enforcement personnel, they should be so informed. Notification should be conducted with compassion. Prior to departing the residence, the medics should provide the next of kin any telephone numbers so that additional questions can be answered and further assistance rendered, if necessary.

When a critically injured person is transported to a hospital, it is recommended that the hospital staff promptly notify the appropriate law enforcement agency. Generally, if the injured person dies shortly after arriving at the hospital, the investigating law enforcement officers should assume responsibility for notifying the survivors of the death.

This is the most difficult part of being a paramedic, hands down. So what do we do? How do we prepare? And why don't we have formal training in this subject?

▨ Have a Plan

It's awkward to be in a position of authority on a scene and not be able to answer questions. Know what your agency protocols are for out-of-hospital death and have a general idea of what your regional policies are for what comes next. Do the police come? Is there an investigation? Who moves the body? Where is the morgue or funeral home? In New York (Suffolk County to be specific), if a paramedic determines the patient meets the criteria for obvious death, then the police officer on-scene will make the notification to the medical examiner. The medical examiner will respond and confirm the death, whether it is due to an illness or by criminal means. The patient is then transported to the medical examiner's office (morgue) by that division. Paramedics technically do not pronounce; we make a presumptive diagnosis of death. Ultimately, the doctor signing the death certificate is the person who makes the absolute decision of death. One way to alleviate some of the family's anguish and eliminate the process of going to the morgue is if a patient has an extensive medical history and the police do not find any obvious signs of foul play, the police will contact the patient's primary physician. If the physician agrees to accept the responsibility of signing the death certificate, then the officer will make a verbal agreement with that physician to sign the certificate of death. In turn, the patient's family can then arrange for a funeral home to pick the body up. Thus, it is extremely important to understand these policies when dealing with "DOA" calls.

▨ *Introduce Yourself*

Introducing yourself rehumanizes the uniform, serving as a small buffer to the information you're about to deliver. It also validates your information as coming from someone in authority, as well as giving the recipient a focal point for questions.

▨ *Identify the Key Players*

Figure out the relationship of those present to the deceased. If possible, try to give the same information to all the adults present at the same time; it will simplify things for them later. Consider segregating small children before speaking; their needs are different and are usually better met through adult family members. When asking the question "Are you the parents/husband/ wife of so and so?" always use the present tense. Referring to the deceased in the past tense can incite confusion and even anger; the information is just too new and has not been processed yet.

Fire the Warning Shot

This is called the "prep statement." It gives the person time to prepare, even on a subconscious level, for the bad news that is coming. In many instances, the person already knows on some level what you are about to say but has not acknowledged it as reality yet. Giving the person a brief review of events gives his or her psyche a moment or two in which to take that proverbial deep breath and prepare itself to process what you're about to say. If you are doing a field pronouncement post-care, an example might be, "We arrived to find your father unconscious. He was not breathing, and there was no pulse, so we immediately began CPR." Do not include large amounts of detail; they will simply not be processed.

Get to the Point

This is called the "core statement." Make the information simple, keep it direct, and try to deliver it with compassion. Using the word "died" or "dead" is important; there is a certainty to the terminology that helps survivors recognize what's going on. You may have to repeat things a few times. The person's psyche will filter out what he or she can't handle; it may take several attempts to get through.

Express Empathy

Empathy is a powerful communication skill that is often misunderstood and underused. Initially, empathy was referred to as "bedside manner"; now, however, educators consider empathetic communication a teachable, learnable skill that has perceptible benefits for both paramedic and patient: Appropriate use of empathy as a communication tool facilitates the interview, increases the efficiency of gathering information, and honors the patient, whether they are alive or dead. Avoid the use of euphemisms. They can confuse and even anger stressed family members. Don't say, "He's in a better place," because you don't know that. Don't say, "I know how you feel," because you don't. Remember that sometimes, less is more.

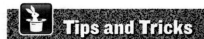 **Tips and Tricks**

HARMFUL PHRASES: BASIC INSENSITIVITY

I know how you feel. My _____ died last year.

We all have to deal with loss.

At least he or she died in their sleep.

He or she had a very full life.

Everything is going to be okay.

Be Prepared for the Aftermath

You have no way of knowing what somebody's grief response might be, and there is no hard and fast rule saying what it should be. You may find that they accept the information tearfully, but rationally, or they may begin rending their shirts, pulling their hair, and keening in ululations of grief. Some may need their hands held; some may need to be pulled away from the deceased. Remember that we are an increasingly diverse society, and although some of this reaction is certainly emotional, there may be a cultural component as well.

In some instances, there may be a significant physiologic reaction. You may be suddenly faced with a person suffering a syncopal episode or other clinical expressions of stress, such as chest pain or respiratory distress. Just because the cause is emotional does not mean it cannot cause the body to go into shock—that is something to keep in the back of your mind as you're tending to the family on scene.

Answer Honestly

This is neither the time nor the place to play crime scene investigator. Don't assume or surmise on facts surrounding the death unless you are certain of the answer and will not be contradicted later on. A dishonest answer on scene may be revealed in other venues, for example, via autopsy, investigations, or future court proceedings. It not only damages your credibility but can cause irreparable harm to the family and shake their faith in the entire agency you represent.

Give Real Information

Know or at least have an idea of what happens next in the process. After survivors weather the first emotional barrage, there are plenty more to come, and often they frankly just don't know what to do next. This is where you can be of enormous help. Just by outlining what the next few steps typically are, you will give them some sort of structure within which to function while trying to sort everything out. If your department supports it, give out supplemental information on support groups or hotlines for grief counseling. Someone may pick up that slip of paper a week later and be grateful for somewhere to turn.

Turn Care Over to Someone Else of Authority

We are just the first in a long line of authority figures survivors will have to deal with. Very often we are the only anchors they can rely on while they try to find some immediate footing. However, we are not designed to be there long term. When you've finished with your role and it's time to leave, make sure you do not leave them without a next contact point. This may be the police officers on the scene or a hospice worker or staff nurse at an extended-care facility, but give them a source for additional questions. Do not leave them without someone to turn to.

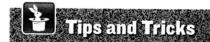

Tips and Tricks

Here are a few additional points to consider:

- Be sensitive and open to families and allow them to express grief and anger. However, be sure to protect your personal safety at all times. I have always taught providers to keep a two-arms-length distance when delivering the news.

- Expect many, many questions. If you don't know the answers to all of them, it's perfectly correct to say, "I don't know, but I will try to get you an answer." It's imperative that you do not speculate on any answers whatsoever.

- Offer simple gestures to the family, such as making any needed phone calls, transporting them to the hospital, or helping to arrange any immediate childcare.

- Be sensitive to the diversity of family structures and the different ways certain cultures choose to express their grief. Individuals need to be treated with dignity and respect regardless of their family structure (domestic partner, common-law spouse, etc.) or culture.

CHAPTER 6

PATIENT SAFETY

"Primum non nocere." ("First, do no harm.")

Emergency Medical Services (EMS) is an important part of the healthcare system and has the responsibility to "do no harm."

The goal of every emergency medical provider (first responder, EMT, paramedic) is to respond to patients in their time of need and to provide them with the most appropriate and highest quality care possible. This care is frequently critical to a patient's health or survival and is often provided in settings that are challenging, chaotic, and even hazardous. Decisions and actions by emergency medical providers are sometimes influenced by environmental factors but are always based on the experience, training, protocols, medical direction, common medical practice, and ultimately the provider's *best judgment*. Regardless of training, experience, and especially the intent of the provider, medical errors in the EMS setting occur and cause harm or even take the life of the very patients the system is intending to save.

As a new paramedic, or salty one at that, EMS providers should be committed to providing a safe environment for all of our patients. Current EMS standards focus on a number of key topics:

- Providing high-quality EMS, including communications and call taking, preparing for arrival, assessing the incident scene, assessing and treating the patient, transporting the patient, and transfer
- Preventing infections and minimizing exposure to hazards
- Ensuring safe operation of EMS vehicles, equipment, and medical devices

- Increasing community awareness of EMS and establishing strong partnerships for public education and emergency preparedness
- Building a high-performing EMS team, including medical oversight, interdisciplinary teams, and work-life balance
- Maintaining user-friendly and effective clinical and information systems for all patients and calls
- Monitoring quality and safety and achieving positive outcomes through data collection and the use of quality indicators
- Reducing the number of infections related to the use of catheters placed in blood vessels
- Patient advocacy
- Paramedics must be consistent with the very highest standards of ethics and integrity. This includes respecting and protecting the privacy rights of our patients. For more information, please read Privacy Practices and Understanding HIPAA (Health Insurance Portability and Accountability Act).

So why is there such a large emphasis on safety? Safety encompasses many areas in EMS. We are directly responsible for the safe delivery of a patient from his or her home, work, street, etc. to the emergency department in inherently dangerous situations. In addition, we are directly responsible for patient confidentiality and we must, and I mean *must*, be an advocate for each one of them. When a person summons EMS, whether we feel it is an emergency or not, as healthcare providers, we must understand, not ridicule or dismiss, why we were called. If we put ourselves in the same position the patient is in, or maybe put your mother, father, grandparent, or child's face in that patient's predicament, would you like someone dismissing their emergency or maybe being disrespectful? I don't think so. If you treat everyone with respect and allow patients to be in control of their dignity regardless of who they are, it will make your job that much easier.

 Tips and Tricks

Patient Advocacy is a concept that most people think they understand, but in all reality, they probably don't really comprehend the scope of it. As an advocate, the paramedic must at times represent the patient, speak for the patient, protect the patient, ensure that the patient is treated appropriately, and ensure that the best decisions are made for the patient and his or her family throughout our interaction with them.

Working as a new medic, I had the misfortune of working with a partner who would ridicule patients because they called EMS if it wasn't a "real" Advanced Life Support (ALS) call. My partner would lambaste the patient, saying he or she was wasting resources, actually making some patients apologize for calling 911. Uncomfortable, to say the least, and if this wasn't bad enough, this partner would do this in the patient's home. As mobile healthcare professionals, we must remember that we are visitors in the patient's home. It was uncomfortable, unsafe, and really not cool. Unacceptable, to say the least! I would spend most of the trip apologizing for the actions of my partner.

Great medics know their place and suck it up when they have to. Someone who smiles and laughs with the upper respiratory infection patient who called 911 at 2 a.m. for a ride to the emergency department. Great medics are willing to sweat buckets while their patient shivers under blankets with the heat cranked up. Great paramedics know when to move quickly and when to relax. I think it has to do little with the shirt we wear off-duty, or our hobbies, or our marital or religious status, or the books we read late into the night, but more about wiping our feet at the front door, introducing ourselves with a smile, and wearing a collared shirt and looking professional when someone calls, no matter the reason. Even if it is to adjust the volume on the TV! Smile, ask if there is anything else we can do to help, then go home and learn how we can better help that person, rather than he or she calling 911. Great paramedics, or EMTs for that matter, know where work and play diverge and can do both to their full extent.

Taking It to the Streets

Before I was in EMS—I think I was around 14 years old—I had a personal experience that made me go into EMS early in life and make me who I am today. I am the oldest of four boys; we shared two bedrooms. My youngest brother was in bed sleeping when my middle brother yelled downstairs to my parents, "Mom, Dad, Danny isn't breathing right!" My father frantically ran up the stairs. I believe he actually stepped on only three steps in the process. He rolled my brother over to find him cyanotic and apneic. He carried my brother downstairs, yelling for my mother to call 911. At first, my father thought he was having a febrile seizure. But, as all three brothers stood there and watched, my father began frantically doing mouth to mouth. I remember very vividly my mother hysterical on the phone as the 911 operator was relaying CPR instructions to her.

My father yelled for me to go outside and flag down the fire department. Well, the fire department arrived within a few minutes. The local volunteer fire department arrived and began resuscitating him on our dining room floor. As my whole family watched them resuscitate him, the ALS provider working on my brother turned around and yelled at my father for lighting a cigarette. He lit a cigarette out of nervousness. You have to understand my father; he rarely shows any emotion, and he was a Vietnam Veteran. And at the time, he was a chain smoker. You know the type. Well, the medics get a pulse and blood pressure on him and prepare to transport him.

Later on that night, my little brother winds up being transferred from the community hospital to which EMS transported him to a hospital that had the resources to take care of him. He ultimately improved over weeks of ICU care and is now 31 years old. Unbelievable, but if you asked my father about the medic who worked on my brother, he to this day has nothing good to say about him. This hatred, still to this day, was from the incident where he was scolded by the paramedic that night. So the moral of the story is "people recall how we treat them respectfully, with kindness, or how poorly we communicate with them and rarely do they remember how we make a difference." Most complaints made by patients are not patient care related. They are poor bedside manner or poor communication skills between EMS and the patient or family.

Now I didn't take anything from the altercation between my father and the medic. What I remember is how they saved my brother's life. This devastating event, directly or indirectly, carved a path for me in the EMS profession—mentally, of course!

TO ERR IS HUMAN

It would be naive to think either that errors in EMS don't exist or that nothing can be done to reduce or even eliminate them. According to an Institute of Medicine report entitled "To Err Is Human" in 2000, there was an estimated 44,000 to 98,000 deaths a year due to errors in medicine.[1] With the emergency department having the highest rate of errors,

---

1   Starfield B. Is US Health Really the Best in the World? *JAMA*. 2000;284(4):483–485.

where does EMS fall? Ten years later, there are no changes. Why? Is the goal to eliminate error, no? Human error cannot be eliminated. It is futile and misdirects resources and causes what our current culture is now: the big wall of "blame and secrecy." Our main goal as new and old EMS professionals should be to reduce harm. If errors are inevitable, how do we improve safety? That is definitely a loaded question. Our current culture in EMS dictates that it is bad to make a mistake. One major way of reducing errors should be to train as you do in the field. We are seeing a lot of simulation labs being utilized in EMS training, which allows us to actually perform skills, hone them, and correct errors before they may happen. That is definitely a great way to teach and train paramedics with all levels of experience.

So by now you must be saying to yourself, why did I decide to go through this? As if medic school wasn't tough enough. The reality is EMS is rapidly progressing into a profession that has undertaken an enormous responsibility. As our healthcare system is at a breaking point, EMS has become a huge stop-gap in many areas of medicine. With new responsibility come a lot of major changes, for the most part good, solid, responsible changes. Think about medic school; how long did you spend on the topic of errors? Did your instructor explain what to do if there is an error, who to report it to, why it is important to be honest, or maybe what our major responsibility as a paramedic is? Probably not!

When I review ambulance and unusual occurrence reports, I find that many different types of errors are made as we care for patients. Fortunately, errors do not happen every day and not all errors result in harm to the patient; however, you also have to wonder how many errors are made that we never catch? The most important thing to remember is that most errors are preventable.

Some common errors in EMS that have resulted in legal action across the nation are as follows:

- Delays in patient care because of an inability to find the patient's location
- Equipment that doesn't work or a lack of knowledge on the provider's part of how it works
- Medication errors
- Esophageal intubation
- Vehicle crashes
- Refusal of care against medical advice of a patient that is not competent

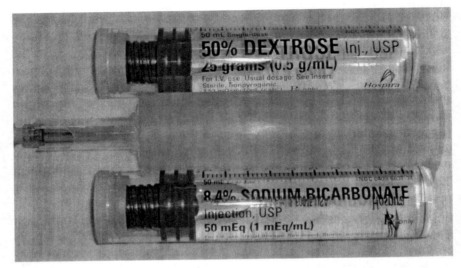

FIGURE 6-1. Photograph of the medications dextrose 50% and sodium bicarbonate 8.4%. Both medications are packaged similarly, are the same size, and fit the same medication shooter. To eliminate the possibility of an error by grabbing the wrong medication, perform the six rights of medication administration every time. Another way would be to set up your medication bag so that the two similar types of medications are not in the same pouch or box. *(Used with permission from Peter A. DiPrima, Jr.)*

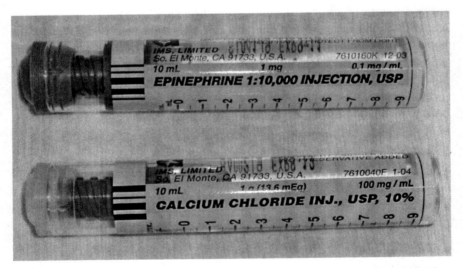

FIGURE 6-2. Two very different medications, same size, and fit the same shooter. Read the label! Perform the six rights of medication administration: the right medication, the right route, the right time, the right patient, the right dose, and the right documentation. *(Used with permission from Peter A. DiPrima, Jr.)*

What can we do as EMS providers to prevent errors?

- Look at your map book and know traffic patterns for different times of the day. If you can't find a location, call dispatch early and get help.

- Occupy your downtime productively: Having nothing to do can produce boredom or anticipation. Both boredom and anticipation are exhausting, and exhaustion can lead to errors.

- Check your vehicle and all of your equipment before you start your shift: Is everything there? Does it work? Do you know how to use it? If you have questions about equipment, ask a supervisor or the education department.

- Maintain your knowledge base and competency: Attend the monthly Continuing Education (CE) programs, subscribe to journals, research current trends on the internet, and use your education money to attend conferences. Check your mailbox for updates and changes in protocols and equipment.

- Always use the five rights when giving a medication (right patient, right drug, right dose, right time, and right route). Don't rely on the fact that every medication container will always be in the same spot in your med box; look at the label and the strength every single time you give a medication. Verify patient medication allergies; check medication name on package; check medication name on container (syringe, vial, ampule, and bottle); check/validate expiration dates; check total container quantity; draw the correct dosage; and verify the drawn dosage. If you are uncertain about a drip calculation or a dosage calculation, have your partner check and verify your math. Don't ever give a medication that someone else has drawn up.

- Use multiple methods of confirming tube placement but always rely on the best: $ETCO_2$. Secure the tube well, continuously monitor the patient's cardiac and Spo_2 status, and immobilize the patient so the patient doesn't dislodge the tube. Frequently reassess your tube and patient, and recheck tube placement after every patient move.

- Take care of yourself and your partner: Fatigue, hunger, thirst, illness, preoccupation, and complacency can all lead to errors. It is your responsibility to know when you can no longer perform optimally.

- Document all of the aspects of competency and capability of the patient to make the decision to refuse care. This is one protocol you should know inside and out, and never skimp on documentation. You want to document each of the seven points in the protocol, and if the patient refuses to sign or walks away, be sure you document that action. Before allowing any patient to sign Against Medical Advice (AMA) be sure you have checked for and documented any possible organic reason for his refusal or that would make him or her incompetent to sign AMA (hypoglycemia, intoxication, dementia, head injury, hypotension, etc.)

- Work as a team: Teamwork can decrease the incidence of certain types of errors. Acting alone or without support can lead to patient care problems on a number or levels.

- Communication is key to making positive differences: Confirm medication orders, reaffirm protocols, and repeat information back to the patient to be sure it was heard correctly. If you are ever unsure of your treatment or want further advice with a patient, don't hesitate to contact a base station physician.

Any error of any magnitude should be reported. Reporting an error immediately protects you and the organization. Sentinel events are errors that have a higher likelihood of causing harm to a patient, attracting media coverage, going up the chain of command as a complaint, or ending in litigation against the organization and/or the care provider. Oh yeah, one other word of wisdom: Never, ever lie! If something occurred or something went wrong during patient care, always tell the truth. Lying can forever change your career in the health profession. There is great trust between EMS employers and their employees. After all, we do carry controlled substances, medications, and drive around in a quarter-million-dollar stocked vehicle. If they can't trust you, they won't want you working for them. I know of a few incidents where a paramedic and his or her partner lied during an investigation and ultimately lost their jobs, not because of the incident that occurred, but because the paramedic lied and tried to cover up what happened. We are human, and errors occur. In EMS, we are forced to make split-second decisions during the most unstable times. Errors occur, but reducing their incidence is our goal.

? Did You Know?

Driving Safely, Arriving Alive!

According to the Centers for Disease Control and Prevention, the number of deaths per 100,000 people in EMS operations is now approaching the number in fire service operations. The rate for EMS providers is now 12.7 deaths per 100,000 workers; the fire service rate is 13.5. The causes of EMS fatalities include electrocution and needle sticks (4%), homicide (9%), cardiac event (11%), and the overwhelming transportation accident (74%).[2]

2 Centers for Disease Control and Prevention. NIOSH Research Leads to a Reduction in Safety Hazards Among Ambulance Service Workers and EMS Responders. U.S. Department of Health and Human Services Publication No. 2010-164. Oct. 2010.

There is a misconception that a larger vehicle may be more dangerous. (An example would be driving a fire truck.) Although that is true when the physics of an accident are applied, the miles placed on an ambulance and the increased frequency of response place it at risk more often. A patient onboard may distract the driver and facilitate riskier behavior. So what are we really doing to focus on ambulance operations? The Emergency Vehicle Operations Course (EVOC) has been around for many years; however, it and programs like it aren't often used for ambulance operations. EVOC highlights how to react to a skid and other defensive driving techniques. New technology using the SKIDCAR system teaches drivers how to avoid getting into a skid, that is, avoiding skidding in the first place. Some training centers have placed ambulances and fire trucks on the SKIDCAR platform to simulate control techniques and skid avoidance. Other techniques and procedures, such as recovering from blowouts, overcorrections, and icy road conditions, also can be simulated in a much smaller space.

By now you should be an experienced EMS provider, new as a paramedic, but not new to the EMS system itself. Do you know that less than half of EMS workers use restraints in the patient compartment! No, I am not talking about restraints for the combative patient; I mean seatbelts for us and the patients we transport. I am sure some of the readers of this book are included in these statistics. But why is that? We respond to some of the most horrific accidents involving non-restrained occupants of motor vehicles, yet we still do not protect ourselves or our patients. Yeah, you could probably say it is uncomfortable, restrictive, or the lap-belt restraint systems commonly provided in patient compartments do not allow full access to the patient. The real issue, however, is that when properly used, the squad bench lap belts position the EMS worker against the side wall, making it impossible for the worker to bend forward to access the patient. If the EMS worker needs to access the cabinets along the driver-side wall, the belts must be unbuckled to allow the worker to stand up. If CPR or other procedures such as intubation or insertion of IVs must be performed, EMS personnel might need to stand over or kneel near the cot. For these reasons, EMS workers often ride unrestrained, seated on the edge of the squad bench. I would be lying if I told you I wore my seatbelt every time, but sometimes we are our own worst enemy. In addition, unrestrained or improperly restrained patients who become airborne in a crash might pose an additional injury risk to EMS personnel and to themselves.

We are responsible for the safety of ourselves, our patients, the public, and other emergency workers when we operate an emergency vehicle. So why are so many ambulances getting into accidents? Emergency operations in EMS are always decisions that are made at the time of each response. Today, Emergency Medical Dispatch, industry data, EMS educational materials, legal case precedents, and other industry practices set a standard of care for emergency vehicle operation that is binding on all EMS providers. Drivers of emergency vehicles are reminded that they solely bear the responsibility for driving safely and with due regard. There is no immunity from liability provided in motor vehicle law for driving. Operating a vehicle in emergency mode is one of the most dangerous activities a prehospital care provider is routinely involved in. Careful consideration must always be given for the lives and safety of the driver, the crew, the patient, and every other person that the vehicle will encounter during the call.

CHAPTER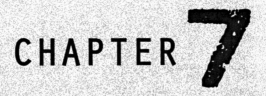

SCENE SAFETY

"BSI, Scene Safety" Poof! You're safe, right! Not really. *Why are so many EMS professionals getting injured or killed at scenes?*

Today, EMT and paramedic students are taught "Scene Safe, BSI" as if it is a protective mantra. I am not convinced that repeating that over and over again makes us any safer. What truly makes us safer is having a realistic appreciation of the real risks of our work and placing logical workplace controls.

One word—SAFETY—includes but is not limited to the safety of you, your partners, your patients, and bystanders. I know you want to ask, isn't medic school over? I had enough learning for a while; why do I have to learn more about this subject? Is this going to be one of those long-drawn-out CME lectures or chapters. No answer! Then why continue to talk about this subject over and over? This is where I open your eyes. If you look in any major EMS trade magazine or journal, take a glance at how many EMS personnel are being injured or killed: not one every month, or every week, but one every day!

Did You Know?

The study entitled "Occupational Fatalities in Emergency Medical Services: A Hidden Crisis" was a peer-reviewed journal of the American College of Emergency Physicians. It documents between 1992 and 1997 that 114 EMTs and paramedics were killed on the job, more than half of them in ambulance crashes. That's an estimated 12.7 fatalities per 100,000 EMS workers, making it close to the death rates for police (14.2) and firefighters (16.5) in the same time period. It's also more than twice the national average for all workers (5.0). Of the 114 deaths, 67 were from ground transportation accidents; 19 from air ambulance crashes; 13 from heart attacks, strokes, and other cardiovascular problems; 10 from homicides, most of them shootings; and 5 from other causes, such as needle sticks, electrocution, and drowning.

If that doesn't open your eyes, when I read this for the first time I said "Holy @#$%".

WHAT IS SCENE SAFETY?

So what is scene safety? Are EMS providers taking appropriate precautions and fully aware of potential hazards on every scene? Any scene has a potential for violence, and many have not-so-obvious indicators of danger. Just as we proceed as if all our patients have blood-borne pathogens, we should respect all patients as having the ability to become violent, cause an unsafe situation, or intentionally injure someone.

Personal safety should be your primary concern on every call, regardless of the call's acuity. Our goals on every call are patient compliance and scene control, both of which directly affect safety. Safety awareness is something that should be applied to every aspect of each call, from dispatch through completion. In this chapter, we focus on applying safety awareness to every patient approach and assessment.

You should always have at least two ways to call for help. Usually paramedics carry a portable radio and a cell phone. Make sure the dispatcher knows that you arrived on the scene. Ask yourself, are there any known dangers? Have the police arrived yet? Has there been any known violence? Is this address "flagged" as dangerous in the dispatcher system? If you are separated from your partner, what is your "Rally Point?"

We exist inside a box of physical space. In normal life, we walk from one safe box to another without really worrying about it, but as a paramedic, it is very easy (if you're not careful) to walk into dangerous boxes and find yourself in peril.

Self-Control = Scene Control

People copy emotions

Keep your voice down

Control your tone

Know your temper level and your partner's

Never run on an emergency scene

Scene Approach: Limit Noise

- Remove loose objects from pockets
- Limit "jingling" equipment
- Do not kick gravel
- Turn radios down to lowest volume where you can hear
- Upon arrival, drive past scene
- Evaluate the scene as you approach
- When parking the vehicle, make sure you can view three sides of the structure
- Do not
  - Park immediately in front of structures
  - Park in driveways
  - Take an unexpected approach
  - Cross yard rather than walkway
- Do not walk next to your partner
  - Spread out
  - Create two targets
- Knock on the door standing on the doorknob side in line with the door frame
- Identify yourself

- Wait for occupant to open the door
- Note whether there are weapons present—obvious and not so obvious

▓ Vehicle Approach: Look for Danger Signs

- No one in vehicle turns around
- Everyone gets out of vehicle, and starts toward you
- "Unconscious person" in properly parked vehicle
- Danger signs
  - Driver adjusts mirrors
    - to watch you
    - to keep lights out of vehicle
  - Persons in vehicle appear to be grabbing or hiding items
  - Vehicle occupants are "out of place"
  - Visible signs of violence—arguing, fighting
  - Dimly lit area

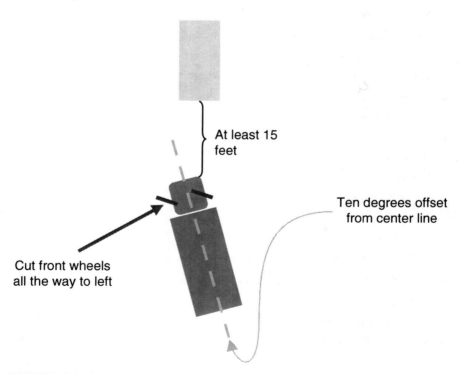

FIGURE 7-I. Vehicle approach.

- Limited access, exit
- "Gut feeling" something is wrong

You must maintain an acute awareness of the structure that surrounds you, the safety of the environment in that structure, and the danger posed by other creatures that might be lingering in there with you. First, you must be careful about the structures—the boxes—you enter. Let's take a car accident for instance: Is gas leaking? Were the airbags deployed? Watch out for broken glass and exposed metal because they create more hazards than you might realize. And speaking of cars, it's easy to become dangerously casual about walking around in traffic. Always be vigilant around moving cars. They're big and they hurt.

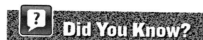

Did You Know?

On November 24, 2008, a provision in the *Manual on Uniform Traffic Control* (MUTCD), administered by the Federal Highway Administration (FHWA), went into effect requiring public safety officers, including volunteer firefighters and EMS personnel responding to an incident on the side of a federal aid highway, to wear a safety vest that meets the Performance Class II or III requirements of the American National Standards Institute/International Safety Equipment Association (ANSI/ISEA) 107-2004 publication.

Minimum requirements for ANSI/ISEA-compliant garments include use of fluorescent yellow-green, orange-red, or red background material with 360-degree retroflective visibility. Garments should be labeled as compliant with ANSI/ISEA 107-2004 or ANSI/ISEA 207-2006.

Second, you must be careful about the safety of the environment *inside* any "box" you go into. Fires produce dangerous gasses like carbon monoxide, low-oxygen environments, and cyanide gas. Be careful of temperature and weather extremes. You can dehydrate at fires or freeze in prolonged extrications in the winter, and lightning can strike you just as lethally as anyone else, whether you're wearing a uniform or not.

When I trained as a probationary volunteer firefighter, we had a training scenario in which everyone in the pool was found floating face down. Bystanders told us that it happened at the exact same time. Of course, all of the "probies" (including me) jumped right in to "save" the swimmers. Our instructor immediately ended the scenario and told us we were all dead. Why? Live electricity in the pool!

There's a basic rule of scene safety that this illustrates: If everyone "in the box" is sick, you will be too if you go in. The consequence to that is that if everyone "in the box" is dead, then you probably will be too if you go in. So, bottom line is don't go in. Sometimes you will have to make a difficult decision, whether to stand outside that dangerous box watching people suffer inside. It's tempting to run in and be the hero, but that can prove deadly. There are people that love you and are waiting for you to come home, and people who are going to have an emergency tomorrow who need you to be there on duty for them.

Your responsibility as a paramedic is to ensure *your* safety, the safety of your partner, the safety of other emergency workers, the safety of your patient, and the safety of any bystanders. In that order! Remember, too, that sometimes "the box" isn't dangerous when you enter it, but the actions you begin to take in the box can make it become dangerous. Releasing oxygen into an enclosed space or defibrillating in wet environments can create dangers that weren't there when you walked in.

Finally, once you've determined that the box you're about to walk into isn't filled with dangerous gas or substances, and that nothing you do in that box is going to risk your safety, you have to start thinking about the other creatures who are in the box with you. People can be dangerous—not everyone is happy to see you, and crowds don't think about who they are hurting. Observe everyone at the scene for body language, be aware of actual or potential weapons that can be used against you, and always keep a clear escape route. Never let yourself become trapped, and always stay with your partner.

🚶 Taking It to the Streets

While operating in the South Bronx, New York, in the early to mid-1990s, I can recall an incident that my partner and I encountered. We responded to a "DIFFBR" call type. In the computer text, it stated that there was a 60-something-year-old female complaining of chest pain and shortness of breath. When we arrived, we saw a few parked cars with broken windows in front of the building. My partner and I looked at each other, and we both decided to get out of there until the police arrived. Just as we were pulling away to a secure area, a young adult ran up to my window and asked where we were going, "My mom is having a heart attack!" We both looked at each other and knew it wouldn't be good. We parked, took our equipment out of the ambulance "bus," and entered the first floor apartment. Oh, did I mention to you that the lobby windows were broken as well. We called dispatch and asked for the police to respond as we were flagged down by the male bystander. As we entered the apartment, I saw an elderly woman in her late 60s sitting on the couch in obvious distress, complaining of crushing chest pain, and shortness of breath. I approached her and sat beside her, introduced myself, and began my assessment. I began taking baseline vitals as my partner attached the ECG electrodes to her. This was before EMS was using 12-leads. To be exact, we were using the LIFEPAK 5. I administered 1/150th grain nitroglycerin sublingual and aspirin, 325 mg PO. She tells us that the pain is still intense, as if there were a "belt tightening around her chest." As we continued to treat her, my partner and I kept looking around the apartment, trying to put the pieces together because this poor woman was so emotional. She tells us that her two sons were fighting over drugs (crack cocaine). Her one son was tired of his brother stealing and always being high. The incident escalated and the brother, who was high, pointed a gun and began shooting at his brother, hence, all the broken glass when we pulled up. Now, my "Spidey" senses are really in overdrive. I look to my partner and say that we need to get her on the chair and to the bus. Just as I got the words out of my mouth, guess who shows up. I'll give you one hint! It wasn't the police. It was the high-on-crack-cocaine brother, who had it in his head as he entered the apartment that no one was helping his mother. Now my partner and I are in a real pickle. We know this guy had a gun. What the heck do we do? It gets even better. We tried to calm him down, but the scene intensified. He became more aggressive and agitated and pulled out a fairly large knife (looked like a hunting knife). He placed it at my stomach and says, "If you don't help my mom, I am going to kill you!" For a split second, I thought about grabbing the knife and doing the unthinkable. But, I decided instead to key up my portable radio and say my unit number over the air and repeatedly state "put the knife down" over the radio for everyone to hear. Thank God the dispatcher knew my voice and called a 10-13 for us. This is the code over the radio for an EMS unit in trouble. It sends out other EMS units and the police department to our location to assist in the situation. Well, I wasn't stabbed, and neither was my partner. We transported the patient to the hospital, who by the way was diagnosed with an inferior wall myocardial infarction. The moral of this story is, if at any time your sixth sense makes you feel uncomfortable, leave. Come back after the police have secured the scene. I came very close to being an assault victim. For the aggressor of this incident, he was arrested and prosecuted for numerous offenses. I was lucky. And luck doesn't always happen.

▨ Never Let Anyone Get Between You and the Way Out

Another basic rule of paramedic scene safety is to consider all family pets have the intent to kill you. Make sure family pets are locked up before you enter. Ideally, the dispatcher will have asked the family to do this, but if it hasn't been done, make sure it gets done quickly.

Ensure your biological safety, ensure the scene safety and then enter 'the box' your patient is in. Now you're ready to ask your first question. What do you think that should be? ...

WHY WAS EMS SUMMONED?

Once your biological and physical safety is ensured (to the best of your ability) and you know what your dispatcher has told you the call is for, you're ready to begin to enter the box and meet your patient.

As you do, take note of the scene as you walk in. What's going on? Is this a car accident? Does the patient look short of breath? How old or young does the patient look? What other clues can you get about the patient just from looking at the environment? Is there home oxygen? Are there asthma inhalers or cigarettes? What can you see? What do you hear? What do you smell? After looking at environmental clues, you then have a decision to make: Is this a trauma or a medical call?

Trauma versus medical is the big decision you need to make at this point. There are a few reasons that you will want to figure this out before you go into a call. The first reason is so that you can anticipate and mentally prepare for what you might encounter. The second reason is that you normally don't carry trauma equipment into medical calls. It's heavy and bulky, so unless you think you'll need it, you leave it in the ambulance (backboards are really big). The third reason is that priorities are different for each situation and different questions are asked.

▨ Trauma Calls

On trauma calls, you want to find out what happened during the accident; when the accident happened—just now or hours or days ago; who was hit; whether there was more than one person; what they were hit with—a car, stick, or pipe. You get the point. These types of questions tell us the "mechanism of injury."

Trauma calls are those that involve accidents. Some examples include the following:

- Car accidents
- Shootings

- Assault
- Stabbing
- Falls causing injury
- Crush injuries
- Animal attacks
- Burn injuries

In automobile accidents, there is list of questions you want to know. For example, was the patient the driver or the passenger? Which seat was the patient in? Was the patient wearing a seatbelt? Were there other passengers in the car who were unrestrained (that could have flown into your patient during the accident)? Were airbags deployed? Did the car roll over? Where was the car struck? In which direction were the two vehicles traveling, and how fast were they going? Was their intrusion into the passenger's compartment? These are all important questions. At the same time, you have to wonder whether the patient might have hurt his or her cervical spine (C-spine).

Medical Calls

On the other hand, if it's a medical call, you need to start thinking about what could have caused the patient to become sick. We call this the "Nature of Illness." Thus, a call for chest pain could mean a heart attack or collapsed lung. An unconscious patient could be due to a stroke, low blood sugar, or seizures. Shortness of breath could be due to asthma, an allergic reaction, or carbon monoxide poisoning.

Medical calls are those that involve someone getting sick somehow. Some examples include the following:

- Heart attacks
- Allergic reactions
- Strokes
- Asthma
- Diabetes
- Seizures
- Poisonings and overdose

Never, ever let your guard down. In January 2009, an Upstate, New York, EMT along with two other EMTs were at a residence treating a 25-year-old man who became agitated and retrieved a high-powered rifle from the bedroom of the residence. As the EMTs were retreating from the residence, the patient (a.k.a., Perpetrator) fired two rounds, one at the victim (i.e., the EMT) striking and killing him.

Understanding what we are responding to helps us mentally prepare for the call and anticipate what we might find. As you become more experienced as a paramedic, you will develop a much longer list in your head of possible causes for the call information you are given. You will also learn how to quickly figure out what is actually going on with your patient when you get there. Later on in the call, when you are exploring the chief complaint and the incident history, you'll learn how to generate a list of potential causes and then how to narrow down the possibilities, but considering the Mechanism of Injury (MOI) or Nature of Illness (NOI) is our first step in answering the question, what is going on? For now, we'll keep it simple. When you are entering a call, think about the MOI or NOI. What should you expect to find? What seems to be going on? What's the incident?

So, what comes next?

WHO'S THERE?

We all hate it when we can't find things. Not finding a patient is a hundred times worse. Before you allow yourself to get too involved in the care of a single patient, you have to ensure that there isn't anyone else on scene that you haven't discovered. The very important next step after determining what happened is to figure out how many patients are there.

When we go into a scene, we are usually dealing with one patient at a time. In a pinch, a medic crew can usually handle two patients, as long as they are not both critically ill. However, if you have more than one critically ill patient or more than two patients all together, you have a multicasualty incident. When that's the case, you have to call for additional help. So knowing how many patients there are, and having a rough idea of how sick they are is an important early step in handling an EMS call. Be aware that there might be more patients than you can initially see when you first walk into the call.

In trauma calls, especially in car accidents, be sure to search around the accident for patients that might have been thrown clear of the cars or for pedestrians that might have been struck and thrown. Remember, improperly restrained babies can travel a long way; they can also get jammed under car seats or pinned in the metal of the car. Patients who are confused may wander away from the scene. Be sure to examine scenes for clues that someone might be missing. If there's a car seat and diaper bag, where's the baby? If there is a purse, where's the woman who owns it? Just because there is a purse or car seat doesn't mean that there has to have been a woman or baby in the car, but it certainly means you should at least check. Bystanders who aren't used to seeing blood can pass out watching you take care of someone who is horribly injured. So be sure to keep an eye on any "crowd" that gathers around you to make sure you don't suddenly have further, unexpected patients.

Also, it's not uncommon for people to be so upset by their loved ones getting sick that they start to get sick too. I responded to one call where a man was having a heart attack, and this was so distressing for his wife that she ended up having a stroke while we were there. These things happen, so when you walk into the scene, make sure you know how many patients you are dealing with before taking your next steps.

SOMETIMES THE HELPERS NEED HELP

People call us when their lives are falling apart and the situation has gotten beyond their ability to cope. Although there is a lot that paramedics can do that the general public can't, we can't do it all. Good rescuers know when they need help, what help they need, and how to get that help to arrive quickly and safely to the right place. Obviously, the first thing you need to know before you call for help is where on earth you are. Usually, this isn't a problem because we call our dispatchers to get help to us, and they should know where we are. However, if you are not where your dispatcher thinks you are, you need to let him or her know that. You also need to let him or her know the best way to get to the scene (access) and the best way to leave the scene (egress). Remember, you can call for help at any time. In fact, medics often ensure that help is requested as soon as we hear the dispatch update (ie, asking for police to attend to a big fight). Sometimes we call for help as soon as we see what we are getting into, and sometimes we only realize half-way through a call that we need some help (ie, when we realize that we are walking into a meth lab). No matter when you realize you need help, as soon as you realize it, call for help immediately. There are two good rules to remember when it comes to calling for help:

1. Stay calm

2. Give precise information

The final thing you need to know when you're calling for help is, what help is out there? The folks you'll call the most are usually the police, the fire department, and of course, other paramedics. The police help control traffic, they control crime scenes, they are the most credible legal witnesses to what happens on a scene, and they are the wonderful men and women who step up when someone tries to hurt us—often at great risk to themselves. The fire department helps contain hazardous materials, secure unsafe structures, and fight fires, and they often get our patients and bring them to us when the environment is too dangerous for us. Other medics can help us to deliver patient care, especially if they have higher levels of medical training than we do. They can help with lifting or by providing an extra pair of skilled hands.

Calling for helicopter medical evacuation is often a good idea in remote areas where our land transport times are more than an hour or so. Some EMS systems have arrangements with their local hospitals to mobilize on-site physician teams for patients who are trapped but need care beyond the paramedic scope of practice.

Don't forget to call your EMS supervisor when necessary; supervisors are an often overlooked resource. Some patients change their mind and decide that they don't want your help, yet they won't sign your refusal form. Other patients just seem like the types that are going to lodge a complaint regardless of what you do. Yet other patients will listen to supervisors more than they will to you, just because they know that they are talking to "the boss." Your supervisor can also help by providing an authoritative legal witness to ensure that you fulfilled your professional duties and obligations to the best of your ability.

Any dangerous animals (I mean just about every animal) should be handled by the experts; call the folks at Animal Control.

Patients with needs that go beyond medical needs can be helped by social service agencies. Dangerous environments often require specialty teams. Some possible sources of help you can call on include the following:

- Hazardous material teams
- Tactical police and paramedic teams
- Marine and diving teams
- High- and low-angle rescue teams
- Enclosed space, and trench rescue teams
- Search and rescue teams (wilderness and urban)
- Vehicle extrication teams
- Disaster response teams

Know which teams are in your area and what their abilities are. If your service doesn't have a lot of information about these teams, this is a great opportunity to invite them in to do a "show and tell" for you as part of your continuing education. Know how to contact public utility crews as well. Electrical crews, natural gas crews, and water crews are all available to help you if you need them. Know who can help you, and know how to call them. Then, when you are in need, send for help.

TALKING TO THE PATIENT

You are about to talk to your patient for the first time and to put your hands on them as well. I'm going to assume that you know all about how paramedics work in teams. As humans, we have a fragile design flaw: We have a huge head, attached by a thin column to the rest of our body—our neck. This means that whenever a strong force pushes our heads or pushes our bodies, there is a danger of our necks being injured or broken. In medical language, we refer to our necks as the "cervical" portion of our spinal column, and we always shorten this to "C-spine." (We don't say "necks"; if you do, you'll sound like a rookie.)

The problem with our necks—I mean our C-spine—is that if they are broken and we move them, we risk breaking them more and injuring our spinal cord, which runs in a column inside our cervical spine bones. If we injure our spinal cord too much, we might become paralyzed, even to the point of losing the ability to breathe on our own. This means that as a rescuer, we have to take exceptionally gentle care of anyone who is (as we say) a possible C-spine injury.

At this point in the call, for the first time we are actually engaging with the patient and speaking to him or her, so it is quite common for the very first words we say to be "please do not move" or "don't turn your head" even before we introduce ourselves. If the MOI suggests a possible C-spine injury, then we have to protect the C-spine of the patient. Now what? At this point, we're getting the first good look at the patient and are trying to get a general impression about who he or she is and how he or she is doing. So now we are ready to form our general impression, which is pretty cool because now we are ready to assess and treat.

What we, as paramedics, have learned through experience is that if you want to paint a clear picture of an incident in another person's imagination, you'll need to include five very specific pieces of information, in the following order:

- The location you are at
- Whether the patient is male or female
- Roughly how old the patient is
- The position you found the patient in
- The level of distress the patient seems to be in

You have to memorize these points, to learn to look specifically for these pieces of information when you approach a patient, and then to report these points, in order, whenever you are presenting your general impression to another medical professional. For example, imagine that there is another, more advanced paramedic crew responding to back you up and they are asking for the general impression of your patient. Imagine that I tell them that I am on the scene with a person in a car accident. Can you form a picture of that in your head?

You might wonder how you can determine a patient's level of distress just by looking at him or her. At this point, it's very, very general. If the patient seems to be fine, is walking around calmly, sitting in a relaxed way, or doesn't look panicked, you can guess (just for now) that he or she is in mild distress. On the other hand, if the patient is collapsed on the ground, is clearly not responding to the environment, or looks as if he or she is in shock or has been really smashed up, then you can guess that the patient is in severe distress. Unless the patient falls in either extreme, we label them as being in "moderate" distress until we find out more. Make sure you're still safe! Are there any threats? This reminds you to pick your head up at this point and just make sure that there aren't any obvious environmental threats to you or your patient that you might have missed or that might have appeared while you were doing your quick assessments. The kinds of threats we worry about are things such as traffic, people, animals, structural damage—almost anything. Basically, you're taking a quick survey of the scene again to ensure that you're not in danger. Then take a quick look at your patient to ensure that he or she is still the way you thought he or she was. Again, you're just performing a quick check to ensure that no new danger is present. After you've done that, you're ready to move on to the ABCs.

Oh yeah, did you make sure you're still safe?

CHAPTER 8

A DAY IN THE LIFE OF A PARAMEDIC

"How are you with blood, vomit, or feces?" This is the first question my partner asks a civilian riding along with him for the day. He is obviously comfortable with it, as he sits inside the ambulance at the beginning of his shift checking the stock of various medications, bandages, IV catheters, and syringes used to draw blood.

"If you're going to get out and be sick, let us know so we don't leave you behind," he says. The Saturday 8 a.m. to 4 p.m. shift will include two seizure patients, a myocardial infarction, almost an hour of *The Wedding Crashers*, and a car accident.

Despite the sensitive care we give to patients inside the ambulance, we seem to dissociate once we transfer the patient to hospital staff. Although professionals say that dissociation is not the healthiest option, paramedics adopt it as part of their job.

"There's not much closure in this job. When you ask how the patient is, it's usually too early to know," says an experienced paramedic. "You see stuff you don't want to see, and it will always stay with you." He adds, "It helps to have attention deficit disorder." Perhaps this defense mechanism keeps us going.

I ask my partner what he thinks about the inherent dangers of this job. He shrugs dismissively and says, "You can't think about it. You just go. You're out there for the patients." For the record, most medics dismiss notions that they worry about death and danger on the job. They say gawkers at accident sites or "psych"(iatric) calls put them in the most danger.

CALL #1

"Not feelin' so well today?" my partner asks gently as he squats before a tall, thin man sitting inside a local homeless shelter at 9:30 a.m., the first call of the day. The man thinks he had a seizure the night before and describes seeing lights and not being able to move. Through further questioning, my medic partner learns the man has a history of mental illness.

The patient feels well enough to walk, so we take him into the emergency department on foot. My partner relays the medical information to the triage nurse, and having transferred care to the hospital, we leave.

■ In the Emergency Room

As my partner writes up the paperwork from the previous call, he hears another medic ask, "What happened to you?" as a tall, bald medic with tattoos streaming up both arms walks into the room. He's wearing white coveralls over his navy paramedic uniform that makes him look like a Stay Puft marshmallow man. "Oh, we had an old fella who was on his way out," he says quietly.

The medics grunt sympathetically. All three are silent, respectful for a moment, and then the medic asks the triage nurse to sign his paperwork. My partner calls the dispatch center to advise them that we need time to clean the ambulance before accepting another call. Our patient has scabies.

■ While Walking Out to the Ambulance Bay...

"Could you pass me a basin and some tissue, please?" asks the tired-looking nurse. A very pregnant patient, who was airlifted to the hospital last night after being pinned beneath a rolled vehicle, lies in the ambulance, with her arm bandaged from fingers to shoulder. It's shortly after 11 a.m. and she's being transported to another hospital for reconstructive arm surgery. The movement of the ambulance makes her nauseated.

Her nurse and the medic sit on the bench beside the stretcher. The nurse comforts the patient as she begins heaving. The medic readies more tissues and says softly, "It won't be much longer now, almost there." The medics then wheel her up to the surgery ward, transfer her to the hospital bed, and leave.

CALL #2

"What's going on here? How come no one called me? Where did this happen?" The mall manager is frantic at the sight of medics in his mall. We ignore him and help the frighteningly pale elderly man off a bench and onto the stretcher. It's 1:30 p.m. and our half-eaten lunches are stashed in the front of the ambulance.

My partner straps an oxygen mask onto the patient while asking questions. I begin placing heart-monitoring electrodes on his chest and print a reading from a tiny monitor stashed under the stretcher. My partner continues to speak loudly to the patient, apparently trying to remain upbeat. The patient's terrified daughter stands a few feet away, watching.

As my partner and I are muttering numbers, almost like a code, back and forth to each other, we check his pulse and monitor his heart. The mall manager still shouts questions and we ignore his intrusion as we focus on our priority: the patient.

We buckle him onto the stretcher, and my partner explains to his daughter that we think her father is having a heart attack, and that she can come in the ambulance or meet us at the hospital. As we wheel the man into the ambulance, my partner is nearly shouting at him, calling his first name, asking what day it is, and how many fingers he's holding up. I jump in the front of the ambulance and calmly flip on the lights and sirens. A pedestrian stares, and his dog howls to the moan of the siren. Road traffic magnetically pulls over to the right (in a perfect world). I floor it through red lights and onto the wrong side of the road. The patient is almost without vital signs. I see my partner in the rear-view mirror piggybacking a dopamine drip. He yells out, "He is in cardiogenic shock." I pick up the pace and race through several stop signs to the ambulance entrance of the hospital.

As we lean over at odd angles and lift the orange blanket under the patient to transfer him to the hospital bed, a young nurse appears and chats with the patient as she looks for a vein to begin a second IV. Her tone changes when she gets no response and shouts, "Sir? Can you hear me?"

A dark-haired nurse with dark circles under her eyes shouts, "Does anyone have any scissors? We need to get his clothes off!" My partner and I help the nurses undress the patient. A doctor in green scrubs runs in. And we bring the hospital staff up to speed on his condition. Another nurse pulls a pastel curtain around the area to guard the patient's privacy. A few seconds later, my partner and I emerge. We fill out paperwork and don't stop to check on the patient on our way out.

Now we are trying to head back to the station.

"Should I?" My partner's fingers hover over the lights and siren switches on the dashboard of the ambulance. A black Toyota sedan comes to a dead stop in the middle of the one-lane road for the fourth time in 100 feet. The driver is clearly confused about where he is going. As medics we are clearly annoyed about his confusion.

My paramedic partner mutters something about temptation. Both of us laugh as the driver turns into a parking lot. We continue back to the station, where we watch movies until our next call.

"So, what are you up to tonight?"

CALL #3

Its 3:20 p.m. and my partner chats with a 20-something passenger of a smashed-up car. She smiles, looks up at him, and giggles, perhaps smitten with his good looks or perhaps because of her head wound from a car accident. Blood runs out of a tiny cut near her temple, turning her blond hair into sticky-looking clumps.

My partner doesn't like what he hears: The woman plans to spend the evening home alone and she has had five drinks in four hours. The young woman's male "friend" rubs her shoulder in a way that makes him feel uncomfortable about leaving her in this man's care. Although she is not seriously injured, we transport her to the hospital for observation.

CALL #4

It's 3:59 p.m. We are dispatched to a "seizure" call at a local homeless shelter. The same shelter we responded to in the morning. As we arrive, my partner and I find our patient lying on the couch in the lobby. The patient quickly begins to shake and twitch—entertaining, but definitely not a seizure. My partner asks the shelter staff about the situation. I respond, "Man, I don't know." The patient looks up at us still shaking and says, "Can't you see I'm having a seizure?" Off to the hospital we go.

BACK AT THE STATION

"What else did we use today?" asks my partner. He restocks the ambulance cabinets at the end of the shift.

The next crew of medics arrives for the Saturday evening shift, generally a busier one because of weekend celebrations. I hand over the keys, and my partner hands over the controlled substances. Another slow night! Both of us head home; neither of us will think about today. It's the only way we can do it all over again tomorrow.

SELF-RESPONSIBILITY

The only person who may really care about you is your mother, but your mother can't wipe your nose forever. When you run into a problem, who are you gonna call? Ghostbusters? There is only one person on this planet that you should rely on—you, yourself. So by now you have to be asking yourself why this topic is discussed in a chapter called "The Day in the Life of a Paramedic." The changing landscape of EMS has been very good, but there also has been a bad side that I hope you will not get yourself caught up in. What does "yourself" mean? It is your very own self. Your self is your innermost being; it's you right here and now. It is the part of you that dreams your dreams. It is the part of you that decides your attitudes. It is the part of you that determines whether you are going to act or react or not act at all. It is what you look at in the mirror every day. It is your body, but it is also your soul. Everything that happens to you is determined by yourself. The sooner you decide what your self is going to be, the sooner you will be able to start setting your goals to succeed in life. Who are you? Who do you want to become? Why?

There are two great, yet conflicting, philosophies of life. Some spend their lives doing the least they can to get by, whereas others spend their lives doing the most they can to get by. There are many advantages to each philosophy; however, only one of these philosophies can ever lead to long-term success. It doesn't take a genius to realize that following the least or slacker mentality will ultimately get you nowhere. People are slackers for many reasons: laziness, victimhood, fear of failure, lack of purpose, or lack of a proper role model. Regardless of the reason, the result is usually the same: lack of long-term success. L-A-Z-Y: There is no excuse for laziness. Lazy people just don't get it. Nothing in this world happens by itself. Things happen because you either do something or don't do something. Remember, for every action, there is a consequence. In EMS, your responsibility as a paramedic has significantly increased. This is not only toward yourself, but also toward your patients. Think about all of those lazy people you may know. Heck, you may have been one yourself. Now is the time to change. Learning is the ultimate act of self-responsibility. Only you gain from learning something. If you are going to base your life on what goes on in a TV sitcom, you're going to be very disappointed. Real life is 24/7/365. When you take responsibility for finding a solution, you own that problem. No one is born smart. Everyone must learn to become smart.

By now, I hope you understand that taking responsibility for your actions and not being lazy is probably the biggest teaching service I can convey to "new" paramedics. After all, you will not be new forever.

CHAPTER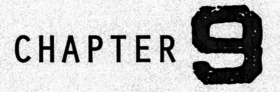

ONE-YEAR ANNIVERSARY

TAKING CARE OF YOURSELF PHYSICALLY AND MENTALLY

Nearly all emergency personnel, EMTs and paramedics included, eventually suffer from a phenomenon known as "burnout," and it is not unusual for personnel to last around 5 years before the stress becomes almost intolerable. Burnout is defined as "exhaustion of physical or emotional strength or motivation usually as a result of prolonged stress or frustration." The key here is the stress is prolonged, typically over a period of several months, and the stress manifests itself through an individual's key life areas, such as psychological, physical, work, and family. It is common to see effects in more than one area simultaneously.

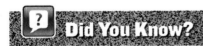 **Did You Know?**

Burnout is a gradual process by which people detach from meaningful relationships in response to prolonged stress and physical, mental, and emotional strain. The result is a feeling of being drained, unproductive, and having nothing more to give.

Emergency personnel suffer very high levels of this type of burnout, and it has been the subject of considerable research. The research has shown that emergency personnel are subjected to five unique stressors:

1. The level of uncertainty is high. When EMTs or paramedics go to work, they have no idea what to expect. It could be a fatal road accident or a serious industrial injury. Most other professions have at least some idea of what they will face when they arrive at work.

2. The sounding of an emergency alarm produces a physical response, and the body prepares itself for the event. Physiological responses include heightened blood sugar levels and increased adrenaline level, blood pressure, and heart rate. These are likely to remain high for several hours, and it's possible that another emergency may occur before the reaction to the first emergency has subsided.

3. The level of interpersonal tension is also high. Emergency personnel work in a crisis environment, and this increases the tension between people to a greater degree than a non-crisis environment. Effects that would be benign in an everyday situation become of vital importance in the theater of an emergency.

4. The exposure to human tragedy is frequent. Whereas most people may never be exposed to a serious emergency situation in their lifetime, emergency personnel can be exposed on a weekly or even daily basis.

5. The fear factor can be extreme. Emergency situations are often frightening, and emergency personnel are expected to deal with both the fear and the situation itself. The increase in legislative action against them if they make what is perceived to be a mistake can also add to the pressure faced by the emergency worker. Added to this is the amount of strain involved in trying to uphold a perceived image.

Once you examine these five stressors, it is easy to see why emergency personnel suffer high levels of burnout, and most cope with it for a low number of years before seeking a route out, by way of either promotion away from the front line or a change in career.

Relaxation Exercise

- Find a quiet place and stretch your whole body. Then, sit down in a comfortable chair where you will not be disturbed. It is best to uncross your legs and rest your hands on your lap, separately.

- Close your eyes. Take a deep breath and blow it out. Repeat.
- Move your feet and ankles and then allow them to relax. Pause.
- Move your knees and lower legs and then allow them to relax. Pause.
- Move your thighs and hip joints and then allow them to relax. Pause.
- Take a deep abdominal breath. Blow it out and relax. Pause.
- Move your shoulders and upper arms and then allow them to relax. Pause.
- Move your forearms and hands and then allow them to relax. Pause.
- Take a deep breath. Blow it out and relax. Pause.
- Notice you can feel your heartbeat at the tip of each finger. Relax and enjoy.
- Move your head and neck and then relax. Pause.
- Move and then allow your jaw, cheeks, forehead, and scalp to relax.
- Remain in this state of relaxation for up to 15 minutes.
- Open your eyes and slowly rejoin the wakeful world, relaxed and refreshed.

SAVING A CAREER BY MANAGING THE DIFFICULTIES

So can burnout be avoided? Research has examined this in some detail, and it is clear that recognizing the stress early and managing it are key. There are some well-known and obvious symptoms to look for: irritability, fatigue, anxiety attacks, and loss of appetite or weight gain due to lack of exercise or overeating. Less obvious symptoms include an increasing reliance on alcohol and tobacco, insomnia, and a general inability to concentrate.

Many departments across the country have implemented a physical fitness program, including medical evaluation to assess the most effective program for an individual. The facts are proven that regular workouts reduce stress, but they are insufficient alone without other forms of support. Stress questionnaires have also proven effective in recognizing the early signs of paramedic burnout, sometimes before any obvious physical signs are apparent. Such questionnaires should be properly designed, confidential, voluntary, and nonpunitive to be properly effective. The stressors are divided into what the department can and cannot control.

Another method that has been found to be effective is education of the sources of stress and self-help techniques to reduce the effects. All of this flies in the face of traditionalists who demand that the profession should stay tough, but effective programs can reduce stress-related deaths and alcohol and substance abuse, and also significantly reduce sick leave and low productivity. The more advanced emergency departments are changing the old mentality of "asking for help is a sign of weakness" to one of real systematic support with real measurable benefits. It is this type of employee assistance program that contributes to reducing burnout as an expectation in the emergency services.

It seems that most people who accept challenges, become good at their craft, and take particular pride in a job well done have difficulty coping with times when they are not 100% successful. However, experiencing "failure" in an EMS role can be haunting. Why? In many cases, lives are literally hanging in the balance, and "the one that got away" could very well be someone's life. Sometimes everything goes right with your patient—you identify the problem quickly, get the IV on the first try, and intubate them without difficulty—and the outcome might still be bad. When resuscitation efforts don't go smoothly, the subsequent feelings of guilt are compounded. Self-recrimination is just one of the stresses of working in the EMS field. Most positions involve long hours, low pay relative to responsibilities, irregular eating and sleeping habits, dealing with difficult patients, managing budget cutbacks, and numerous other challenges—all in a setting where one slipup can result in death or disability to patients who are depending on you to never make a mistake. And that's not to mention the many potentially traumatizing scenes that EMS workers are exposed to: the suicide patients, pediatric traumas, child abuse cases, assault and rape victims, and a host of other upsetting and tragic situations that the average citizen may go an entire lifetime not encountering.

The greatest problem we have in EMS is that no matter how well we train, the concept of dealing with death is never fully understood. In EMS, people die, and sometimes there is nothing we can do about it. Being in a relatively new emergency service (paramedicine), there is no uniform way to deal with death and other stresses of our job. Are we healthcare providers? The answer is unequivocally yes. So if we address critical stress, we have to be approached with the same critical stress as physicians and nurses do. However, our particular brand of stress differs from that of nurses and doctors. To add a little statistical information to a stressful topic, according to psychologytoday.com, there are 300 to 400 physician suicides each year, the most of any profession.

The question is trying to find what type of stress we may encounter. Are we in stressful situations similar to police officers? Yes. How many times are we shot at, threatened, and assaulted? How many times do we enter the homes of our patients, not knowing what we will encounter in these strange surroundings? Therefore, our particular brand of stress must incorporate debriefing designed in part for law enforcement professionals. Are we often in harm's way similar to firefighters? Again, the answer is yes. Whether it is responding to a motor vehicle accident with lights and sirens, crawling into confined spaces to help a patient in need, or treating the helpless while debris falls around us, our profession involves a fair amount of risk. EMS is an inherently dangerous job.

EMS personnel have been targets during incidents such as the Columbine school shootings, the bombing of the Oklahoma City, Alfred P. Murrah federal building, the 1993 World Trade Center attack, release of gas in the New York City subways, and the attack on September 11, 2001, of the World Trade Center and the Pentagon. EMS personnel are trained to save lives and operate under the EMT Oath taken to preserve life, but EMS personnel now face the uncertainty that police officers and firefighters do, and there is no guarantee of returning home to their families at the end of their shift. Paramedics and EMTs do not carry a firearm. Their only means of safety is a law enforcement presence, and that's still not a safety guarantee.

It is a useful concept to say "scene safety" first. This is actually a great rule of thumb, but if we are not willing to accept risks, then we do not fully understand the magnitude of responsibility entrusted to us by our partners, brothers and sisters in other public service professions, and those who rely on us to do the right thing. Our job is not to fight fires, perform surgery, or treat the wounded in the middle of a firefight. However, the rules of the street sometimes mandate that we do all of these things. Sometimes scene safety is not possible to help save a life. Scene safety is a rule, but sometimes rules need to be broken. Many of our brother and sister EMTs and paramedics have gone above and beyond the call of duty. Let's look back at September 11, 2001, at Paramedic Keith Fairben and EMT Mario Santoro of New York Presbyterian EMS (both of whom I supervised and will never forget), or FDNY Paramedic's Carlos Lillo and Ricardo Quinn, or the other countless rescuers that went above and beyond that day from the World Trade Center, Pentagon, and Shanksville, Pennsylvania. That does not mean those who do not take great risks are without bravery, but it does point out the enormity of responsibility and related stress that we encounter on a daily basis.

EMS STRESS

With all of these different types of risk factors, there has to be a development of a new modality to treat "EMS stress." Once a treatment of "EMS stress" is developed, it has to be implemented uniformly by social workers, psychiatrists, and other mental health professionals who have some clue of what we do every day. The second part of a new treatment modality is how we are educated to deal with this unique stress. Crews need to be put out of service until they are cleared medically to return to work. Every significant event needs to be monitored by a designated health officer who is actively involved in EMS. I am sure that there are some systems that have these protocols in place, but they are rare. Very similar to law enforcement after a police-related shooting occurs, we have to get out of the habit of sending a crew back out to the street after an event that would put the everyday person into therapy for life. After all, we are only human.

In order for us to be able to function in our jobs, we must be able to build an immunity to the loss of life; otherwise, we would be proverbial basket cases. Nevertheless, know it or not, it affects us the same exact way it affects the "average Joe." The only difference is that we can put it into the recesses of our minds and not fall apart at the seams. What happens is that we have the potential to fall apart internally long before we manifest it in our daily lives.

Finally, there must be a balance between what we are able to do to serve the public and what needs to be done to keep coworkers and ourselves on an even keel. The obvious answer is resources. Time, money, and personnel are needed to keep our profession healthy and happy. The time is now to plan. Our state and local councils, in addition to meeting the needs of the patient, must address the long-term effects of EMS stress on its members. It will be decades before the physical and psychological effects are known for those of us who put on a uniform every day and make house calls. It would be ironic if the prehospital professionals of today would be the in-hospital patients of tomorrow.

? Did You Know?

A 2006 article in *Northwest Public Health* states that most studies estimate the prevalence of posttraumatic stress disorder (PTSD) among EMS personnel as ranging from 15% to 20%. Although it may not sound like much, one in five workers with PTSD is a statistic that cannot be ignored. No doubt many other workers suffer from less serious symptoms of stress and anxiety.

These days, large EMS organizations such as hospitals and urban fire departments take measures to help public safety professionals deal with the stress of the job and the toll it can take. Some agencies offer free services such as grief counseling, drug and alcohol abuse prevention and treatment, and even spiritual counseling. Others require employees who've been involved in particularly traumatic events to participate in mandatory Critical Incident Stress Debriefing (CISD) sessions. Smaller agencies may not offer as wide an array of employee services, and even larger ones have been forced to cut back in the slumping economy.

Ultimately, finding coping strategies that work are as personal and individual a process as choosing the right stethoscope or finding a compatible EMS partner. No single solution fits for everyone, but taking steps to modulate the negative effects of stress is imperative, particularly for those wanting to make a career of public safety work. Field-based EMS workers are taught from the first day of training that securing the scene is of paramount importance. As the saying goes, you can't rescue others if you need rescuing yourself. Scene safety usually refers to imminent physical hazards, like downed power lines or a patient with a weapon. However, the same premise applies to the everyday physical and emotional well-being of EMS workers.

Here are a few ideas for managing stress that may help you become a more valuable employee and ultimately a better lifesaver:

- Learn to recognize possible signs of stress and get help if you think you need it. According to the Mayo Clinic website, symptoms of stress may include the following:
  - Physical: headache, back pain, chest pain, heart disease, heart palpitations, high blood pressure, decreased immunity, stomach upset, and sleep problems.
  - Mental and emotional: anxiety, restlessness, worrying, irritability, depression, sadness, anger, feeling insecure, lack of focus, burnout, and forgetfulness.
  - Behavioral: overeating, undereating, angry outbursts, drug or alcohol abuse, increased smoking, social withdrawal, crying spells, and relationship conflicts.

If you do have stress symptoms, taking steps to manage your stress can have numerous health benefits. Stress management can include physical activity, relaxation techniques, meditation, yoga, and Tai-chi. In the internet age, technology also facilitates communicating with colleagues about difficult situations and sharing suggestions for coping strategies. Find a few EMS forums or social media groups that seem interesting and join in the conversation (see Appendix B).

- Take advantage of free employer resources. As noted above, organizations have begun to recognize the toll of stress on public safety workers and have implemented various programs to help. These may include employee assistance programs (EAPs) that provide counseling for workers under stress, access to a gym or workout equipment, an active CISD team, and even spiritual counseling, for example, a fire department or hospital chaplain. Using available time off in the form of paid vacation or mental health days is another way to escape the pressures of the job and return to work feeling refreshed.

- Learn from your mistakes. One of the most difficult parts of working in EMS is that people's lives depend on your actions. However, the truth is that caregivers are not robots, and no one comes out of paramedic or nursing school being perfectly skilled and adept. That is certainly not an excuse for being careless, but even when you try your hardest, the outcome may be less than ideal. Take every opportunity to talk things over with your team members, supervising physician, and others who can share their experiences and wisdom and help you improve your skills and achieve better results. Pursue continuing education and strive to upgrade your diagnostic and technical knowledge and abilities.

- Accept the things you cannot change. Most stress management experts believe that a great deal of stress comes from trying to "control the uncontrollable." Although it is valiant to want to help people—the goal of nearly everyone who pursues an EMS career—the fact is there will always be elements of the job that are beyond your control.

So why am I talking about such depressing topics? After all, you just started in this profession or maybe decided you were getting burned out as an EMT and began looking for another career path within EMS. Whatever the reason, you are the future of this profession and understanding what you are up against reduces job-related stress. I could definitely sit here and write war stories for you, but I would rather you understand that our training is very limited when it comes to the well-being of the paramedic. Remember, this topic was in the first division of medic school, and you probably spent an hour or two on the topic. Perhaps the best coping strategy is simply to revel in your accomplishments (you just went through medical school in 1 year). Focus on the lives you've saved, the patients you've helped, and the colleagues you've taught. Although stress can never be completely eliminated, you can mitigate its effects by managing it before it starts managing you. Be safe, take care of yourself, and seek help when you need it.

CHAPTER 10

WHAT'S NEXT FOR PARAMEDICS?

To many people, the term "paramedic" is synonymous with anyone that may show up with a rescue unit to the aid of those in need. Many simply do not realize that there is a vast difference in education, skill, and responsibility among the varying levels of responders to a scene. A large percentage of people call 911 to request the "paramedics," not knowing that who actually shows up at an emergency scene may be a basic EMT or even a firefighter with only first-responder-level training.

One possible reason for the diluted meaning of "paramedic" in the public eye could be because responders work so well together during an emergency situation. Most emergency units have somewhat illusive lives, even when on duty. Although they may be easy to spot as they travel through cities with sirens blaring and lights flashing, they are typically not the type of people that display rankings or boast their hierarchy to the public. Even if they did display badges, emblems, or insignias that represented their ranking or level of care, most people would not know the meaning. In fact, the only time that it may be obvious who is a higher rank may be during an emergency situation. The problem is, during those types of situations, many people are focused on the problem at hand and not necessarily on who is making decisions.

EMTs, paramedics, firefighters, and first responders of all levels work together in a well-organized harmony during any type of response. Although all responders to a situation clearly know who is making the decisions, it may not be obvious to onlookers, because even high-ranking officials are usually part of the rescue effort, alongside any subordinates.

YOUR CAREER AS A PARAMEDIC

Today's paramedic is a healthcare professional that plays a vital role in emergency care. However, due to the diligence and continued efforts of programs backing paramedics, they are now also stepping up into stronger roles in long-term care of patients. These days, it is not at all uncommon to see paramedics working in emergency departments, intensive care units, and in some cases, even nursing homes. Paramedics are starting to become known in many facets of healthcare and can often be found anywhere the need for emergency care of a patient may come to be.

Paramedics have long since faced the old stigma of being pertinent only in emergency patient care. However, today's paramedic training involves far more than just emergency medicine and may include long-term care for geriatrics and pharmaceuticals that extend far beyond the scope of emergency medicine. Additionally, paramedics today are trained in advanced cardiac care and diagnostics, and even some surgical and orthopedic techniques. The paramedic on the street today has knowledge in virtually all areas of healthcare and has the ability to apply that knowledge in almost any situation.

Paramedics have never stopped seeking education. Through the efforts of support groups and training institutions, the paramedic has been able to continuously receive training that increases their knowledge and skill. Continued education has even become part of a paramedic's requirements for maintaining certification or licensure. Every paramedic is required to attend certain amounts of classroom training each year, just to stay certified.

Proving their dedication to education and their devotion to the healthcare industry, paramedics are actively seeking new pathways in medicine. While some seek education and step into areas of healthcare such as radiology, extended care, and surgery, others actively seek roles in nursing and therapeutic functions. Paramedics are found in educational venues, such as the paramedic to registered nurse online program, and even moving on to medical schools and using their ambition and knowledge to apply themselves in medicine to become physicians.

WHAT HAPPENS TO PREHOSPITAL CARE IF PARAMEDICS CONTINUE TO ADVANCE INTO LONG-TERM CARE?

Because a paramedic, or EMT-P, is actually part of a multitiered program of training, consisting of EMT-Basics, EMT-Advanced, and in some states EMT-Intermediate, it only serves to reason that the lower levels are learning new skills and techniques as well. Many states across the country have already recognized the EMT-I as an active and working prehospital care provider. Knowledge, skills, and techniques once only utilized by paramedics are now being used by these individuals in the field. Techniques typically performed by paramedics, such as advanced cardiac care, intravenous injections, and advanced airway maneuvers, are being performed by EMT-Basics and EMT-Intermediates, bringing some relief to the heavy burden of responsibility that has historically been placed on paramedics alone. Institutions that teach and govern emergency medical responders have recognized the need for alternatives to paramedics in the field. With more and more paramedics leaving "the streets" in search of new fields of study and employment in medicine, other levels of EMTs are being trained to fill the roles once held by the paramedic.

THE FUTURE OF THE PARAMEDIC

Though still somewhat unknown, one thing is certain: Paramedics have proven themselves to be individuals that constantly strive to become better professionals in the healthcare scene. Their diligence has not gone unnoticed, and through their continued efforts and training, they are moving into virtually all areas of healthcare. For more than 40 years now, paramedics have dedicated their lives to serving patients and to building upon the ideas of what a paramedic is to be. They have been extremely successful helping to create a solid emergency medical response system and are now proving their worth in other facets of patient care. A role that was once thought to be a simple ride to the hospital for patients is now patient care within minutes of an incident that continues into days and even years of long-term care for those patients. Paramedics have come a long way since the days of Johnny and Roy. Education has opened doors that were never before available. Accredited college degree programs have been created, allowing paramedics to not only obtain a solid degree in paramedic science, but also to transition into new medical fields. Paramedic to registered nurse programs have paved the way for paramedics to cross over into the nursing field. Some colleges allow credit to paramedic certifications and licenses toward programs such as physician assistant, public personnel management, and even business degree programs.

The role of a paramedic has changed over the years. They are no longer being thought of as just someone that can stop bleeding and rush a patient to the hospital. They are proving themselves as leaders in emergency medicine and students with the capacity to learn advanced studies. By being persistent and continually working toward new career advancements, paramedics have created a whole new pathway into medicine.

APPENDIX A:
STATE EMS AGENCIES

ALABAMA
Office of EMS and Trauma
    Department of Public Health
The RSA Tower
201 Monroe Street, Suite 750
Montgomery, AL 36104
334-206-5383; Fax: 334-206-5260
Website: www.adph.org/ems/

ALASKA
Community Health & EMS Section
DHSS/Public Health
P.O. Box 110616
Juneau, AK 99811-0616
907-465-3027; Fax: 907-465-4101
Website: www.chems.alaska.gov

ARIZONA
Arizona Department of Health Services
150 North 18th Avenue, Suite 540
Phoenix, AZ 85007
602-364-3150; Fax: 602-364-3568
Website: www.hs.state.az.us/bems

ARKANSAS
Division of EMS & Trauma Systems
Arkansas Department of Health
5800 West 10th Street, Suite 800
Little Rock, AR 72204
501-661-2262; Fax: 501-280-4901
Website: www.healthyarkansas.com/ems/

CALIFORNIA
Emergency Medical Services Authority
10901 Gold Center Drive, Suite 400
Rancho Cordova, CA 95670-6073
916- 322-4336; Fax: 916-324-2875
Website: www.emsa.ca.gov

COLORADO
Colorado Department of Public Health
    & Environment, EMS Division
4300 Cherry Creek Drive South,
    HFEMS-A2
Denver, CO 80246-1530
303-692-2980; Fax: 303-691-7720
Website: www.cdphe.state.co.us/em/

CONNECTICUT
Connecticut Department of Public
Health, Office of EMS
410 Capital Avenue, MS#12EMS
Hartford, CT 06134-0308
860-509-7975; Fax: 860-509-7987
Website: www.dph.state.ct.us

DELAWARE
Blue Hen Corporate Center
655 South Bay Road, Suite 4-H
Dover, DE 19901
302-223-1350; Fax: 302-223-1330
Website: www.dhss.delaware.gov/
dph/ems/

DISTRICT OF COLUMBIA
DC Department of Health/
Emergency Health & Medical
Services
64 New York Avenue, NE,
Suite 5000
Washington, DC 20002
202-671-4022; Fax: 202-671-0707
Website: www.bioterrorism.dc.gov

FLORIDA
Florida Department of Health,
Bureau of EMS
4052 Bald Cypress Way, Bin C18
Tallahassee, FL 32399-1738
850-488-0595; Fax: 850-921-6365
Website: www.doh.state.fl.us/mqa/
emt-paramedic/

GEORGIA
Emergency Medical Services
2600 Skyland Drive
Atlanta, GA 30319
404-679-0547; Fax: 404-679-0526
Website: www.ems.ga.gov

HAWAII
State of Hawaii
Department of Commerce and Consumer
Affairs, Professional and Vocational
Licensing Division
Attention: BME
P.O. Box 3469
Honolulu, HI 96801
808-586-2708
Website: http://hawaii.gov/health/
family-child-health/ems/

IDAHO
Idaho Emergency Medical Services
Bureau
650 West State Street, B-17
P.O. Box 83720
Boise, ID 83720-0036
877-554-3367; Fax: 208-334-4015
Email: iadahoems@dhw.idaho.gov

ILLINOIS
Illinois Department of Public Health
525 West Jefferson Street
Springfield, IL 62761-0001
217-782-4977; Fax: 217-782-3987
Website: www.idph.state.il.us/ems/

INDIANA
Indiana Department of Homeland
Security, EMS Certifications
302 West Washington, E239, IGC-S
Indianapolis, IN 46204-2739
317-234-7223; Fax: 317-232-3895
Website: www.in.gov/sema

IOWA
Iowa Department of Public Health
321 East 12th Street
Des Moines, IA 50319-0075
515-281-7689
Website: www.idph.state.ia.us/ems

KANSAS
Kansas Board of Emergency Medical
 Services
Landon State Office Building
900 Southwest Jackson Street, Suite 1031
Topeka, KS 66612-1228
785-296-7296
Website: www.ksbems.org

KENTUCKY
Kentucky Board of Emergency Medical
 Services
300 North Main Street
Versailles, KY 40383
859-256-3565; Fax: 859-256-3128
Website: www.kbems.kctcs.edu

LOUISIANA
Office of Public health
Bureau of Emergency Medical Services
11224 Boardwalk Drive, Suite A1
Baton Rouge, LA 70816
225-275-1644; Fax: 225-275-1826
Website: www.dhh.lousiana.gov/
 offices/?id=220

MAINE
Jay Bradshaw, Director
Maine Emergency Medical Services,
 Department of Public Safety
45 Commerce Drive, Suite #1
152 State House Station
Augusta, ME 04333-0152
207-626-3860; Fax: 207-287-6251
Website: www.maine.gov/dps/ems

MARYLAND
Institute for Emergency Medical
 Services Systems
653 West Pratt Street
Baltimore, MD 21201-1536
410-706-5074; Fax: 410-706-4768
Website: www.miemss.org

MASSACHUSETTS
OEMS
99 Chauncey Street,
 11th floor
Boston, MA 02111
617-753-7300; Fax: 617-753-7320
Website: www.mass.gov/
 dph/oems

MICHIGAN
Michigan EMS Section
P.O. Box 30717
Lansing, MI 48909
517-241-0179
Website: www.michigan.gov/
 mdch

MINNESOTA
MN EMS Regulatory Board
2829 University Avenue SE,
 Suite 310
Minneapolis, MN 55414-3222
800-747-2011; Fax: 651-201-2812
Website: www.emsrb.state.mn.us

MISSISSIPPI
State Department of Health
EMS/Trauma Care System
P.O. Box 1700
Jackson, MS 39215-1700
601-576-7380; Fax: 601-576-7373
Website: www.ems.ms.gov

MISSOURI
Missouri Department of
 Health
Bureau of EMS
P.O. Box 570
Jefferson City, MO 65102-0570
573-751-6356; Fax: 573-751-6348
Website: http://dhss.state.mo.gov/
 ems

MONTANA
EMS & Trauma System Section
Montana Department of Public Health
  & Human Services
P.O. Box 202951
Helena, MT 59620
406-444-3895; Fax: 406-444-1814
Website: www.dphhs.mt.gov/ems

NEBRASKA
Division of Emergency Medical
  Services
301 Centennial Mall South, 3rd Floor
P.O.Box 95026
Lincoln, NE 68509-5007
402-471-0124; Fax: 402-471-0169
Website: www.hhs.state.ne.us/ems/
  emsindex.htm

NEVADA
Nevada State Health Division
4150 Technology Way, Suite 101
Carson City, NV 89706
775-687-7590; Fax: 775-687-7595
Website: www.health.nv.gov/ems_
  emergencymedical.htm

NEW HAMPSHIRE
Bureau of EMS
33 Hazen Drive
Concord, NH 03305-0003
888-827-5367; Fax: 603-271-4567
Website: www.state.nh.us/safety/ems

NEW JERSEY
NJ Department of Health & Senior
  Services
Office of EMS
P.O. Box 360
Trenton, NJ 08625-0360
609-633-7777; Fax: 609-633-7954
Website: www.state.nj.us/health/ems

NEW MEXICO
EMS Bureau, Department
  of Health
P.O. Box 26110
Santa Fe, NM 87502-6110
505-476-7702; Fax: 505-476-7810
Website: www.health.state.nm.us

NEW YORK
Lee Burns, Director Bureau
  of EMS
New York State Health
  Department
433 River Street, Suite 303
Troy, NY 12180-2299
518-402-0996; Fax: 518-402-0985
Website: www.health.state.ny.us

NORTH CAROLINA
Office of EMS
2707 Mail Service Center
Raleigh, NC 27699-2707
919-855-3935; Fax: 919-733-7021
Website: www.ncems.org

NORTH DAKOTA
North Dakota Division of EMS
  and Trauma
600 E. Boulevard Avenue;
  Dept. 301
Bismarck, ND 58505-0200
701-328-2388; Fax: 701-328-1702
Website: www.nd.health.gov/ems

OHIO
Ohio Department of Public Safety,
  Division of EMS
1970 West Broad Street
Columbus, OH 43218-2073
614-466-9447; Fax: 614-995-7012
Website: www.ems.ohio.gov/

OKLAHOMA
State Department of Health, EMS
  Division
1000 Northeast 10th Street,
  Room 1104
Oklahoma City, OK 73117
405-271-4027; Fax: 405-271-4240
Website: www.health.state.ok.us/
  program/ems/

OREGON
EMS & Trauma Systems Section
800 Northeast Oregon Street,
  Suite 465
Portland, OR 97232
971-673-0520; Fax: 971-673-0555
Website: www.oregon.gov/dhs/
  ph/ems

PENNSYLVANIA
Bureau of EMS Office, Pennsylvania
  Department of Health
625 Forster Street
Harrisburg, PA 17120
717-787-8740; Fax: 717-772-0910
Website: www.health.state.pa/ems

RHODE ISLAND
Emergency Medical Services
  Division
3 Capitol Hill, Room 105
Providence, RI 02908
401-222-2401; Fax: 401-222-3352
Website: www.health.state.ri.us/hsr/
  professions/ems/

SOUTH CAROLINA
SC DHEC, Division of EMS
2600 Bull Street
Columbia, SC 29201
803-545-4200; Fax: 803-545-4212
Website: www.scdhec.gov/health/ems/

SOUTH DAKOTA
Emergency Medical Services
118 West Capitol Avenue
Pierre, SD 57501-2000
605-773-3178; Fax: 605-773-3018
Website: www.state.sd.us/dps/ems

TENNESSEE
Division of Emergency Medical
  Services
Heritage Place, Metro Center
227 French Landing, Suite 303
Nashville, TN 37243
615-741-2584; Fax: 615-741-4217
Website: www.state.tn.us/health/ems

TEXAS
EMS & Trauma Systems Coordinator
  Office
Texas Department of State Health
  Services
P.O. Box 149347
Austin, TX 78714-9347
512-834-6700; Fax: 512-834-6736
Website: www.tdh.state.tx.us/hcqs/ems/
  emshome

UTAH
Bureau of EMS, Department
  of Health
Box 142004
Salt Lake City, UT 84114-2004
800-284-1131; Fax: 801-273-4149
Website: www.health.utah.gov/ems/

VERMONT
Emergency Medical Services Division
Department of Health
Box 70, 108 Cherry Street
Burlington, VT 05402
802-863-7310; Fax: 802-863-7577
Website: www.state.vt.us/health/ems

VIRGINIA
Virginia Department of Health
Office of EMS
1041 Technology Park Drive
Glenn Allen, VA 23059
804-888-9100; Fax: 804-371-3108
Website: www.vdh.state.va.us/oems

WASHINGTON
Office of Emergency Medical & Trauma
    Prevention
P.O. Box 47853
Olympia, WA 98504-7853
360-236-4700; Fax: 360-236-2829
Website: www.doh.wa.gov/hsqa/
    emstrauma

WEST VIRGINIA
West Virginia Office of Emergency
    Medical Services
350 Capitol Street, Room 425
Charleston, WV 25301
304-558-3956; Fax: 304-558-1437
Website: www.wvoems.org

WISCONSIN
Bureau of EMS & Injury Prevention,
    DHFS/P.H.
1 West Wilson Street
Madison, WI 53703
608-266-1865;
    Fax: 608-261-6392
Website: www.dhfs.state.wi.us/
    ems

WYOMING
Jim Mayberry, EMS Program
    Manager
Wyoming Department
    of Health
Hathaway Building,
    Room 446
Cheyenne, WY 82002
307-777-7955; Fax: 307-777-5639
Website: www.wdh.state.wy.us/
    sho/ems

APPENDIX B: FEDERALLY SPONSORED EMS PROGRAMS AND FEDERAL AGENCIES

FEDERALLY SPONSORED EMS PROGRAMS

Emergency Medical Services for Children National Resource Center
http://www.childrensnational.org/EMSC/

Healthy People 2010
http://web.health.gov/healthypeople/

HRSA Rural Health Access to Emergency Devices Grant Program
http://ruralhealth.hrsa.gov/funding/aed.htm

HRSA Rural Health Network Development Grant Program
http://ruralhealth.hrsa.gov/funding/network.htm

HRSA Rural Health Outreach Grant Program
http://ruralhealth.hrsa.gov/funding/outreach.htm

HRSA Rural Hospital Flexibility Grant Program
http://ruralhealth.hrsa.gov/funding/flex.htm

HRSA Trauma-EMS Program
http://www.hrsa.gov/trauma/

National Center for Disaster Medicine and Public Health
http://ncdmph.usuhs.edu

FEDERAL AGENCIES

Agency for Healthcare Research and Quality
http://www.ahrq.gov/

Center for Medicare and Medicaid Services
http://www.cms.hhs.gov/

Centers for Disease Control and Prevention (CDC)
http://www.cdc.gov/

Consumer Product Safety Commission
http://www.cpsc.gov/

Department of Health & Human Services
http://www.hhs.gov/

Department of Homeland Security
(DHS)
http://www.dhs.gov/

Department of Justice (DOJ)
http://www.usdoj.gov/

Department of Labor
http://www.dol.gov/

Department of Transportation
http://www.dot.gov/

FDA Medwatch
http://www.fda.gov/medwatch/articles.
htm

Federal Emergency Management
Agency
http://www.fema.gov/

Fire Administration (USFA)
http://www.usfa.dhs.gov/

Food and Drug Administration
http://www.fda.gov/

Health Resources and Services
Administration (HRSA)
http://www.hrsa.gov/

National Center for Health
Statistics
http://www.cdc.gov/nchswww/

National Guideline Clearinghouse
(NGC)
http://www.guideline.gov

National Highway Traffic Safety
Administration (NHTSA)
http://www.nhtsa.dot.gov/

National Institutes of
Health (NIH)
http://www.nih.gov/

National Library of Medicine
http://www.nlm.nih.gov/

Office of Inspector General
http://www.oig.hhs.gov/organization/
OCIG/index.html

Office of Rare Diseases—National
Institutes of Health (NIH)
http://rarediseases.info.nih.gov/
ord/

Trauma.org
http://www.trauma.org/

APPENDIX C: EMS ASSOCIATIONS

EMS ASSOCIATIONS IN THE UNITED STATES

Alabama EMT Association
www.aemtaonline.com

American Ambulance Association
www.the-aaa.org

American Heart Association
www.americanheart.org

Arkansas EMS Association
www.aemta.org

Association of Air Medical
Services
www.aams.org

California Ambulance Association
www.the-caa.org

Delaware State EMS Association
www.dvfassn.com

EMS Association of Colorado
emsac.org

Florida Association of Professional
EMT and Paramedics
www.fapep.org

Georgia Association of EMS
www.ga-ems.com

Idaho EMS Association
www.idahoems.com

Illinois Ambulance
Association
www.illinoisambulance.org

Indiana EMS Association
www.theindianaemsa.org

Iowa EMS Association
www.iemsa.net

Kansas EMS Association
www.kemsa.org

Louisiana Association of National
Registered EMTs
www.laemt.com

Maine Ambulance Association
www.the-maa.org

Michigan Association of EMTs
www.maemt.org

Minnesota Ambulance Association
www.mnems.org

Missouri EMS Association
www.memsa.org

National Association of EMTs
www.naemt.org

National EMS Management
  Association
www.nemsma.org

Nebraska EMS Association
www.nemsa.org

Nevada EMS Association
www.nema-nv.org

New Mexico EMS Association
www.nmemta.org

New York State Volunteer Ambulance
  Association
www.nysvara.org

North Carolina Association of Rescue
  and EMS, Inc.
www.ncarems.org

North Dakota EMS Association
www.ndemsa.org

Ohio Association of EMS
www.oaems.org

Oregon EMS Association
www.oregonems.com

Pennsylvania Emergency Health
  Services Council
www.pehsc.org

South Carolina EMS Association
www.scemsassociation.com

South Dakota EMT Association
www.sdemta.org

Tennessee Ambulance Service
  Association
www.tennesseeambulance.com

United States First Responders
  Association
www.usfra.org

Wisconsin EMS Association
www.wisconsinems.com

Wyoming Association of Pre-hospital
  Providers
www.wyoproviders.org

INTERNATIONAL ASSOCIATIONS
International Association of Chiefs of
  Police
http://www.theiacp.org/

International Association of Emergency
  Managers
http://www.iaem.com/

International Association of Fire Chiefs
http://www.iafc.org/

International Association of Fire
  Fighters
http://www.iaff.org/

International Rescue and Emergency
  Care Association
http://www.ireca.org/ireca/

APPENDIX D: RESOURCES RELATED TO EMS

Advocates for EMS
http://www.advocatesforems.org/

Air & Surface Transport Nurses
Associations
http://www.astna.org/

Air Medical Safety Advisory Council
http://www.amsac.org/

American Academy of Emergency
Medicine
http://www.aaem.org/

American Academy of Pediatrics
http://aap.org/

American Ambulance Association
http://www.the-aaa.org/

American Association of Poison
Control Centers
http://www.1-800-222-1222.info/
poisonhelp.asp

American Burn Association
http://www.ameriburn.org/

American College of Cardiology
http://www.acc.org/

American College of Emergency
Physicians
http://www.acep.org/webportal

American College of Osteopathic
Emergency Physicians
http://www.acoep.org/

American College of Surgeons
http://www.facs.org/

American Health Care
Association
http://www.ahca.org/

American Medical Association
http://www.ama-assn.org/

American Public Health
Association
http://www.apha.org/

American Red Cross
http://www.redcross.org/

American Society of Anesthesiologists
http://www.asahq.org/

American Stroke Association
http://www.strokeassociation.org/

American Trauma Society
http://www.amtrauma.org/

Association of Air Medical Physicians
http://www.ampa.org/

Association of Air Medical Services
http://www.aams.org/

Association of Emergency Physicians
http://www.aep.org/

Association of State and Territorial
Health Officials
http://www.astho.org/

COMCARE Emergency Response
Alliance
http://www.comcare.org/

Commission on Accreditation of
Ambulance Services
http://www.caas.org/

Committee on Accreditation of
Education Programs for the EMS
Professions (CoAEMSP)
http://www.coaemsp.org/

Commission on Accreditation of
Medical Transport Systems
http://www.camts.org/

Continuing Education Coordinating
Board for EMS
http://www.cecbems.org/

Emergency Nurses Association
http://www.ena.org/

Homeland Security Institute
http://www.homelandsecurity.org/

NIMS/NRP Resources from Homeland
Security Institute
Joint Commission on Accreditation of
Healthcare Information
http://www.jointcommission.org/

NAADAC, The Association for
Addiction Professionals
http://naadac.org/

National Association for Search and
Rescue
http://www.nasar.org/nasar/

National Association of Air Medical
Communications Specialists
http://www.amsac.org/

National Association of Counties
http://www.naco.org/

National Association of EMS Educators
(NAEMSE)
http://www.naemse.org/

National Association of EMS
Physicians (NAEMSP)
http://www.naemsp.org/

National Board of Medical Examiners
http://www.nbme.org/

National Center for Emergency
Medicine Informatics
http://www.ncemi.org/

National Collegiate EMS Foundation
http://www.ncemsf.org/

National Emergency Management
Association
http://www.nemaweb.org/

National Emergency Medicine
Association
http://www.nemahealth.org/

National Emergency Number Association
http://www.nena9-1-1.org/

National EMS Information System
http://www.nemsis.org/

National EMS Memorial Service
http://www.nemsms.org/

National EMS Pilots Association
http://www.nemspa.org/

National Patient Safety Foundation
http://www.npsf.org/

National Public Safety
Telecommunications Council
(NPSTC)
www.npstc.org

National Registry of EMTs (NREMT)
http://www.nremt.org/

National Rural Health Association
http://www.nrharural.org/

National Safety Council
http://www.nsc.org/

National Stroke Association
http://www.stroke.org/

National Trauma Bank
http://www.facs.org/trauma/ntdb.html

NIMS/NRP Resources from
Homeland Security Institute—Joint
Commission on Accreditation of
Healthcare Information
http://www.jointcommission.org/

North American Association for
Ambulatory Urgent Care
http://www.nafac.com/

Radiological Society of North America
(RSNA)
http://www.rsna.org/

Raven Maria Blanco
Foundation
http://www.rmbfinc.org/

Society for Academic Emergency
Medicine (SAEM)
http://www.saem.org/

Society of Emergency Medicine
Physician Assistants (SEMPA)
http://www.sempa.org/

Society of Trauma Nurses
http://www.traumanursesoc.org/

Sudden Cardiac Arrest Association
http://www.suddencardiacarrest.org/

Transportation Safety Advancement
Group (TSAG)
http://www.tsag-its.org

Wilderness Medical Society
http://www.wms.org/

APPENDIX E: MENTAL HEALTH AND TREATMENT PROGRAMS

Brattleboro Retreat Mental Health and
 Addiction Retreat
www.brattlebororetreat.org
1-800-738-7328

People who participated in the New
 York City World Trade Center
 rescue, recovery, and cleanup
 operations but who live outside the
 New York City area may be eligible
 for monitoring and treatment
 services funded by the federal
 government with no out-of-pocket
 costs. Call 877-498-2911 for more
 information.

In New Jersey:
Division of State Police and Department
 of Law and Public Safety
Employees can obtain EAP services by
 contacting a 24-hour hotline:
800-FOR-NJSP
800-FOR-NLPS

West Coast Post-Trauma
 Retreat: 415-721-9789

Mental Health America
2000 N. Beauregard Street, 6th Floor
 Alexandria, VA 22311
Phone: 703-684-7722
Fax: 703-684-5968
Toll free: 800-969-6642
TTY Line: 800-433-5959

TREATMENT LOCATORS
Mental Health Services Locator

Phone: 800-789-2647 (English and
 Español)
Phone: 866-889-2647 (TDD)
Website: www.mentalhealth.samhsa.
 gov/databases

*Substance Abuse Treatment Facility
 Locator*

Phone: 800-662-HELP (ext. 4357)
 (toll-free, 24-hour English and
 Español treatment referral
 service)
Phone: 800-487-4889 (TDD)
Website: www.findtreatment.samhsa.gov

HOTLINES

National Suicide Prevention Lifeline

Phone: 800-273-TALK (ext. 8255)

SAMHSA National Helpline

Phone: 800-662-HELP (ext. 4357)
  (English and Español)
Phone: 800-487-4889 (TDD)

Workplace Helpline

Phone: 800-WORKPLACE
  (967-5752)
Website: www.workplace.samhsa.gov/
  helpline/helpline.htm

REFERENCES

1. Strathern P. *A Brief History of Medicine*. New York: Carroll and Graf; 2005.
2. Taylor B. Napoleon's faithful field surgeon. *Military History*. 1997;14(2):46-52.
3. Cooper J, Steel K, Christodoulou J. Mobile coronary care—a controversial innovation. *N Engl J Med*. 1969;281(16):906–907.
4. Rose L, Press E. Cardiac defibrillation by ambulance attendants. *JAMA*. 1972;219(1):63–68.
5. Pantridge J, Geddes J. A mobile intensive care unit in the management of myocardial infarction. *Lancet*. 1967;7510(2):271–273.
6. Moiseev SG. Experience in the administration of first aid to patients with myocardial infarction in Moscow. *Soviet Med*. 1962;26:30–35.
7. National Academy of Sciences; National Research Council. Accidental death and disability: the neglected diseases of modern society. A report of the Committees on Trauma, Shock, and Anesthesia. 1966.
8. Walz B. *Introduction to EMS Systems*. Albany, NY: Delmar; 2002.
9. Public Law 93-154. "Emergency Medical Services Systems Act." Ninety-third United States Congress. Signed November 16, 1973.
10. Emergency Medical Services Amendments. Public Law 94-573. Ninety-fourth U.S. Congress. Signed October 21, 1976.
11. National Academy of Sciences; National Research Council. Emergency medical services at midpassage. A report of the Committee on Emergency Medical Services. 1978.
12. Page J. National Study of Paramedic Law and Policy. 1975–1976. Lakes Area Emergency Medical Services; 1976.
13. Page J. *The Paramedics: An Illustrated History of Paramedics in Their First Decade in the U.S.A.* Morristown, NJ; Backdraft Publications; 1979.

14. Mobile Intensive Care Paramedics. Wedworth-Townsend Act, Article 3. State of California. Signed July 14, 1970.

15. Graf W, Polin S, Paegal B. A community program for emergency cardiac care. *JAMA*. 1973;226(2):156–160.

16. Phoenix Fire Department Emergency Transportation. City of Phoenix—Phoenix Fire Department Website. http://phoenix.gov/fire/etrans.html. Accessed September 12, 2010.

17. San Diego Medical Services Enterprise History. San Diego Medical Services Enterprise Website. http://www.sdmse.com. Accessed September 15, 2010.

18. Davis D, Ochs M, Hoyt D, Marshall L, Rosen P. The San Diego Paramedic Rapid Sequence Intubation Trial: A three year experience. *Academic Emerg Med*. 2003;10(5):446.

19. National Academy of Sciences; National Research Council. *Medical Requirements for Ambulance Design and Equipment*. Washington, DC: National Academy of Sciences; 1968.

20. National Center for Health Services Research; Health Services Research and Evaluation Unit; Department of Health Services Administration. *Community Planning for Emergency Medical Services*. Pittsburgh, PA: Graduate School of Public Health, University of Pittsburgh; October 1977.

21. Eisenberg M. Eugene Nagel and the Miami Paramedic Program. *Resuscitation*. 2003;56:243–246.

22. Nagel E, Hirschman J, Nussenfeld S, Rankin D, Lundblad E. Telemetry-medical command in coronary and other mobile emergency care systems. *JAMA*. 1970;214(2):332–338.

23. Nagel E, Hirschman J, Nussenfeld S. Mobile physician command: a new dimension in civilian telemetry-rescue systems. *JAMA*. 1974;230(2):255–258.

24. Birmingham Regional Emergency Medical Services System Overview. The Birmingham Regional Emergency Medical Services System Website. http://www.bremss.com/overview.htm. Accessed September 9, 2010.

25. Medford R. Obituary for Ralph Feichter. *The Mountaineer*. March 7, 2005.

26. Page J. Volunteers can't do it. *Paramedics Int*. Spring 1976:28–31.

27. Staresinic C. Send Freedom House. *University of Pittsburgh-Pitt Chronicle*. February 23, 2004.

28. Warren J, Hill F, Faehnie L. The Columbus story of mobile emergency care[pamphlet]. Ohio State University, Ohio; Ohio State University Department of Medicine; 1975.

29. Warren J, Lewis R, Stang J, Fulkerson P, Sampson K, Scoles A. Effectiveness of advanced paramedics in a mobile coronary care system. *JAMA*. 1979;241(18):1902–1904.

30. Dodley C. The Columbus Heartmobile Project 1969. *The Siren*. Summer 2005.

31. Sherman M. Mobile intensive care units. *JAMA*. 1979;241(18):1899–1901.

32. Garfield E. Can the new health practitioners reduce medical costs? Part 1: Physician assistants and emergency medical technicians. *Essays: Information Scientist*. 1980;4(13):433–440.

33. Warren J, Lewis R, Stang J, Fulkerson P, Sampson K, Scoles A. Effectiveness of advanced paramedics in a mobile coronary care system. *JAMA*. 1979;241(18):1902–1904.

34. Omnibus Reconciliation Act of 1981. Public Law 97-35. Ninety-seventh U.S. Congress. Signed August 13, 1981.

35. Brennan J, Krohmer J. *Principles of EMS Systems*. Dallas, TX: American College of Emergency Physicians; 2006.

36. Ambulance service in the United States. *J Emerg Med Services*. January 1986:57.

37. Pan American Health Organization. *Emergency Medical Services Systems Development: Lessons Learned from the United States for Developing Countries*. Washington, DC: World Health Organization; 2003.

38. National Academy of Sciences; National Research Council. Injury in America: A Continuing Public Health Problem. Prepared for the U.S. Department of Transportation; 1985.

39. Beauchamp TL, Childress JF. *Principles of Biomedical Ethics*. 2nd ed. New York: Oxford University Press; 1983.

40. Yania v Bigan, 397 US 316 (PA 1959) 155 Atlantic 2d 343 (PA 1959).

41. Miles SH, Crimmins TJ. Orders to limit emergency treatment for an ambulance service in a large metropolitan area. *JAMA*. 1985;254:525–527.

42. American College of Emergency Medicine. Guidelines for Do Not Resuscitate orders in the prehospital setting. *Ann Emerg Med*. 1988;17:1106–1108.

43. Brock DW, Wartman SA. When competent patients make irrational choices. *N Engl J Med*. 1990;322:1595–1599.

INDEX

Page numbers followed by *f* indicate figures.

long spine board. *See* backboard
lung sounds. *See* auscultation

medevac helicopter, 4, 6*t*
medical calls, 99
medical emergencies, 61
medical examiner, 76
medication
    error prevention, 86*f*, 87
    errors, 86*f*
medicines, 15-18
mentor, 30, 63, 65
military
    combat medicine, 33
    conflict, 1
    paramedic training, 35
mini guide, resume writing, 39
mistakes, 118
motor vehicle crashes, 73, 88. *See also*
    ambulance; vehicle approach

Napoleonic Wars, 1
National Academy of Science, 5
National Academy of Sciences'
    Committee of Emergency
    Medical Services, 10-11
National Association of EMTs, 12
National Commission for Certifying
    Agencies, 27
National Highway Safety Act of
    1966, 9
National Highway Traffic Safety
    Administration (NHTSA),
    15-18, 21
National Registry Paramedic, 31
National Research Council, 8-9
nature of illness, 99
needle decompression, 69
needle sticks, 88
NHTSA. *See* National Highway Traffic
    Safety Administration
noise limitation, 93-94
nonemergent calls, 61
non-life-threatening medical
    emergencies, 61

objective
    new personnel resume, 51
    writing, 44-45
occupational fatalities, 92
offshore paramedic, 34-35
opportunities, career, 27-36
organizations, 30

Page, J., 11-12, 11*f*
paramedic, 7. *See also* critical care
    paramedic; dive paramedic
    technician; flight paramedic;
    military; offshore paramedic;
    rig medic; tactical paramedic;
    websites
    day in life of, 106-110
    future, 119-122
    medicines and, 15-18
    military training, 35
    new, tips for, 64-66
    pediatric patients, 15-18
    personal experience calls, 96-97,
        106-108
    personal testimony, 59-66
    roles and responsibilities,
        18-21
    survey questionnaires, 12
    titles for, 12
    training course, 12
paramedic job. *See also* resume; resume
    writing
    obtaining, 37-57
    one-year anniversary, 111-118
    street application, 59-79
paramedicine, 1-14, 114
patient
    advocacy, 24-25, 82
    best interest of, 70
    confidentially, 72
    critically ill, 100-101
    distress, 104
    intubated, 68
    safety, 81-90
    talking to, 103-104
    unconscious, 99